PRAISE FOR

GRETCHEN BECKER'S

THE FIRST YEAR™ –
TYPE 2 DIABETES

"The most practical and useful guide to diabetes that I have ever seen. Gretchen Becker understands how diabetes feels and what diabetics need to know."
—RICHARD PODELL, M.D., M.P.H.,
Clinical Professor, UMDNJ-
Robert Wood Johnson Medical School

"Gretchen Becker explains the realities of diabetes . . . she gives you an 'attitude' for dealing with health care professionals and teaches you to become your own best patient advocate. This is not only a reassuring survival manual for the first year, but a reliable reference book for the rest of your long and happy life with diabetes."
—JUNE BIERMANN AND BARBARA TOOHEY,
founders of Sugarfree Diabetes Centers
and authors of nine books on diabetes,
including the Diabetic's Total Health and Happiness Book

"Wouldn't I have loved to find this book when my doctor told me that I have diabetes! Reading this book during my first year dealing with diabetes would have spared me a lot of anxiety and misunderstanding. Becker tells it like it is. She is completely up-to-date on the science and practice of diabetes and shares her real world experience as an expert who happens to have type 2 diabetes herself. The greatest strength of this book is the wise way in which she deals with the most controversial area of diabetes treatment—what to eat. There is nothing anywhere that comes close to her comprehensive coverage or makes better sense than what you will find here."

—RICK MENDOSA,
diabetes journalist

"I went to my family doctor recently for a routine checkup. Much to my surprise and dismay, he diagnosed type 2 diabetes. My first stop was the bookstore, where I was fortunate to find your book. I took it home and read it over the next few days. I want to thank you for your excellent and encouraging book."
—COLIN PORTNUFF

"I love the book by Gretchen Becker. I just bought it and it has been so very helpful. I'm still really struggling with everything (counting, tracking, choosing, limiting, measuring...I feel like a science experiment!) She makes it all seem possible and not quite so scary. I find that the more I understand something, the better I'm able to cope with it." —JEAN VIGNES

"Your book is wonderful to read. Your personal style is very affecting and your language is clear and careful. You have provided information I never knew; it will be infinitely valuable to your readers. Your humor breaks me up. Just the right amount." —VIRGINIA PAGE

"If you can only buy one book on type 2 diabetes—this is it! Gretchen Becker's book has brought together so much solid information and has achieved the nearly impossible goal of presenting it in a very readable style. After twenty-three years of living with disease, I learned much by reading this book. Thank you, Gretchen." —RHODA MARTIN

"I just had to write you about your book. It is very well written and I am recommending it to my classes and on my local radio program. The information in your book is well organized and your message about guilt is long overdue. I was in public education (elementary) for most of my life and now that I am retired, I am on a mission to teach people to make sensible decisions about lifestyles. I have put your book at the top of the list of recommended readings." —DR. ANDREA TIKTIN-FANTI

"I just wanted to congratulate you on the excellent book you wrote. I particularly liked your approach to the issues regarding eating. For many years I have been involved in the design and development of innovative diabetes education programs and I am glad to see the approach toward dietary management is starting to slowly come around. Thanks again for your excellent contribution!" —TOM CONANT

"The best book for type 2s is The First Year™—Type 2 Diabetes by Gretchen Becker. It is especially good for newly diagnosed diabetics but I recommend it for all type 2s. The organization makes it especially valuable with 'need to know' stuff up front and more detail later." —ROBERT DENNETT

"I got a call from the nurse that my tests showed diabetes and the doctor needed to see me. While waiting the two days for the appointment I went to the bookstore and bought this book. When I saw the doctor I had a better understanding of what he was trying to explain because I had read so much of it already. It helped me know what questions to ask and kept me from being completely overwhelmed by all the information you get at that first treatment plan visit. Since then this book has traveled with me everywhere so it's always close at hand if I need to look something up." —DEBRA CARMICHAEL

STOP DIABETES

ALSO BY GRETCHEN BECKER

The First Year™—Type 2 Diabetes

GRETCHEN BECKER

Foreword by
Allison B. Goldfine, M.D.

STOP
DIABETES

50
**simple steps you can take at any age
to reduce your risk
of type 2 diabetes**

Illustrations by
Virginia Rose Page

MARLOWE & COMPANY
NEW YORK

Published by
Marlowe & Company
An Imprint of Avalon Publishing Group Incorporated
161 William Street, 16th Floor
New York, NY 10038

Library of Congress Cataloging-in-Publication Data

Becker, Gretchen.
Stop diabetes : 50 simple steps you can take at any age
to reduce your risk of type 2 diabetes / by Gretchen Becker.
p. cm.
ISBN 1-56924-563-0 (trade paper)
1. Non-insulin-dependent diabetes—Prevention—
Popular works. I. Title.
RC662.18 .B433 2002
616.4'6205—dc21   2002141441

9   8   7   6   5   4   3   2   1

Designed by Pauline Neuwirth, Neuwirth & Associates
Printed in the United States of America
Distributed by Publishers Group West

To the Whitingham-Jacksonville (Vermont)
Lions Club, whose members care
about diabetes

CONTENTS

Foreword by Allison B. Goldfine, M.D.   xi
Preface   xv
Introduction: Diabetes 101, The Short Course   xvii

1. Eat less and move more   1
2. Learn about the glycemic index   5
3. Don't exercise: Play   11
4. Learn to fill up on high-fiber foods   13
5. Learn to tango   17
6. Avoid trans fats   19
7. Listen to recorded books or music   23
when your workout is routine
8. Learn what processed, or refined, carbohydrates are—   25
and don't overdose on them
9. Understand how diabetes progresses   31
10. Understand that diets are controversial   37
11. Eat real food   43
12. Find something to do at home that's   47
more interesting than TV
13. Understand that starch is sugar   51
14. Learn the symptoms of diabetes   55
15. Don't diet: Be a gourmet   59
16. Start not smoking   63

17. Read ingredients and labels   65
18. Get friendly with a farmers market   71
19. Take your family along   75
20. Keep an eye on your fats and blood pressure   79
21. Learn to waste   81
22. Laugh more   85
23. Lobby for better food choices at work or school   87
24. Get a meter and test after meals   91
25. Enjoy rich food——on special occasions only   95
26. Don't overdo the browned foods   99
27. Go easy on the fruit juice   103
28. Be careful with diet products   105
29. Be a trendsetter   107
30. Eat something red, green, or orange with every meal   111
31. Focus on saving time, not labor   115
32. Carry a doggy box   119
33. Consider weights   123
34. Plant a garden   125
35. Do chores for elderly neighbors   131
36. Get a buddy   133
37. Drink sodas as treats, not all day long   137
38. Learn your heritage   141
39. Make your food more difficult to eat   145
40. Go window-shopping   149
41. Analyze your approach to eating   151
42. Eat more fish   157
43. Discard the idea of *good* and *bad*   161
        in reference to your eating habits
44. Make your meals relaxed and social   163
45. Combine extra calories with extra exertion   167
46. Make sure you're getting essential vitamins and minerals   171
47. Spend more time with little children   173
48. If diet and exercise don't work,
        ask your doctor about medications   175
49. Stay informed   179
50. Be in charge of your destiny   183

        Afterword   185
        Resources   187
        About the Author   193

FOREWORD

By Allison B. Goldfine, M.D.

gretchen becker has been a superb teacher to me over the years that I have had the honor of knowing her. With tremendous insight she has questioned every word of medical advice I have ever offered her, and she has found unique ways to translate the recommendations of her medical team successfully into her daily routine. In her first book, *The First Year—Type 2 Diabetes*, Ms. Becker offered sound and practical advice to improve the health of people with diabetes—especially, but not only, those newly diagnosed. Now, in her second book, she provides guidelines to prevent the development of diabetes in people at risk for the condition.

A brief description of the types of diabetes will help you better understand this book. There are two main kinds of diabetes—type 1 and type 2. In type 1 diabetes, for some reason the body attacks and destroys the pancreatic beta cells, which make insulin. In the absence of these insulin-making cells, and thus insulin, the nutrients in food—and specifically glucose—cannot properly get into the cells of the body and thus be used as a source of energy. In people with type 2 diabetes, there is both a decrease in the relative amount of insulin that the body can make and a decrease in the ability of insulin to act. This reduction in insulin action is termed insulin resistance. This book focuses on the prevention of type 2 diabetes. Insulin resistance is associated with excess weight, high blood pressure, high cholesterol levels, and increased risk of cardiovascular diseases including heart attack or stroke.

Both excess weight and diabetes are epidemic in the United States as well as in western societies. At present there are over 300,000 excess obesity-related deaths each year in the United States alone due to diabetes, stroke, coronary artery disease, and cancer. Although there are clearly genetic (inherited) traits increasing the risk of diabetes and obesity, the marked recent increases in rates of these conditions far exceed the rate of any changes that may be occurring at the level of the genes and must be accounted for in large part by changes in lifestyle. These findings make it critical for Americans to incorporate more healthy lifestyle choices into their daily routines.

New studies demonstrate that people at very high risk for developing diabetes, and who have the most modest increases in blood sugar, can delay or prevent the onset of type 2 diabetes effectively with lifestyle changes or with the initiation of medical therapies. Although drug treatment may appear easier, changes in lifestyle have been shown to be more effective in disease prevention. Also, lifestyle changes do not involve long-term exposure to medicines that may have untoward side effects and complications in the people who take them. Improved food choices (a euphemism for diet) and increased physical activity (exercise) can safely and effectively reduce weight gain and prevent diabetes and the associated complications. The lifestyle changes required to significantly impact on one's health are modest: Ten to twelve pounds of weight loss and thirty minutes of exercise, such as walking, performed five days a week, are sufficient to reduce the risk of development of diabetes by over 50 percent in persons at high risk. No drug therapy will work effectively or make diabetes go away in the absence of these lifestyle changes.

In *Stop Diabetes*, Gretchen Becker presents information on healthier lifestyle choices in a manner that can be incorporated into one's daily life. Practical suggestions from her years with diabetes, and from the experiences of her acquaintances, provide an array of approaches that could work for you or for your loved ones. The advice is sound and presented with humor, a most valuable companion for those seeking to make changes each day for their health.

ALLISON B. GOLDFINE, M.D. is an Assistant Professor at Harvard Medical School, and an Investigator at the Joslin Diabetes Center in Boston. Her research work focuses on understanding insulin resistance and its role in the development of type 2 diabetes and complications. She lives outside of Boston with her husband and three daughters.

PREFACE

having diabetes is no fun. I know. I have type 2 diabetes myself. That's why I'd like to do whatever I can to help other people avoid ever getting this very inconvenient disease.

Once you have type 2 diabetes, your life becomes very restricted. You have to watch every single bite of food that goes into your mouth, because food is what makes your blood sugar levels go up, and high blood sugar levels are what diabetes is all about. You have to cut out sugary, fatty treats almost completely. You even have to limit the amount of starchy foods like potatoes and rice that you can eat.

Once you have type 2 diabetes you can, of course, choose to ignore it, to continue to eat as you always have. But if you do, you're practically guaranteed of getting some of the complications of diabetes, including kidney failure, blindness, and amputated limbs. Also heart attacks. The longer you have diabetes, the more apt you are to get these complications.

Today we are seeing an epidemic of type 2 diabetes, and even children are being diagnosed. Because this means they will face decades with this disease, their probability of eventually developing complications is high.

Rather than risking this bleak future, it's much better if you can act *now* and take steps that will reduce the chances that you will ever develop type 2 diabetes yourself, even if the disease runs in your family. It may mean making a few sacrifices today. But if you can make a few sacrifices today, you may avoid having to make a ton of sacrifices tomorrow.

If I'd known twenty years ago what I know now about diabetes, I would probably not have it today. Since my diagnosis in 1996, I've learned a lot about this disease. I've written a book for the newly diagnosed called *The First Year—Type 2 Diabetes* (Marlowe, 2001). Now I'd like to share some of this information with those who don't yet have diabetes but who think they may be at risk. Please take it seriously. It may save your life.

diabetes 101, the short course

if you're reading this, you probably have a relative with diabetes, or maybe a friend or colleague. You may have seen how difficult it is for this person to manage the disease, and you'd like to do whatever you can to prevent it in others—including yourself.

Congratulations! The best thing you can do to help prevent diabetes is to become informed. The fact that you've taken the trouble to open this book means that you're motivated to make some changes in your life. Sometimes motivation is the most difficult and most important step in a new journey. Now you've taken the first step. So take a deep breath and prepare for the rest of the journey.

Diabetes means too much sugar in the blood

BEFORE YOU CAN learn what you can do to reduce your risks of getting diabetes, you need to understand what diabetes is, what causes it, what risk factors you can change, and what risk factors you cannot.

Basically, diabetes means that the level of sugar in your blood is too high. When I say *sugar* I don't mean table sugar, which scientists call *sucrose*. I mean another sugar called *glucose*. Thus people often refer to *blood glucose*, or sometimes *BG* for short. Sometimes people just say *blood sugar*. It's the same thing.

Everyone has glucose in the blood. You need glucose to provide energy for all the cells in your body. When you have diabetes, you just have too much of a good thing. Your blood sugar is too high.

Why is it too high? Basically, because you have a problem with a hormone called *insulin*. Insulin helps glucose get into the cells to be burned for energy. Without insulin, the glucose can't get into the cells and accumulates in the blood, and the blood glucose levels get higher and higher.

People with type 1 diabetes, which used to be called juvenile diabetes because it usually was diagnosed in children or teenagers, don't produce enough insulin, and they inject insulin to bring their blood glucose levels down. No one knows exactly what causes type 1 diabetes, and at this time there is very little that anyone can do to prevent it, although scientists are finding clues that may lead to preventive steps in the future.

The other kind of diabetes, which this book is about, is type 2 diabetes. People with type 2 diabetes usually produce plenty of insulin, often even more than normal. But they have something called *insulin resistance*, which means that for some yet-unknown reason, their insulin doesn't work very well. People with type 2 diabetes can reduce their insulin resistance and bring their blood glucose levels down with diet, exercise, oral drugs, and sometimes insulin injections as well.

The cause of type 2 diabetes
is not completely understood

IF I COULD tell you exactly what causes type 2 diabetes, I'd be a good candidate for a Nobel Prize. Unfortunately, I can't, which is a shame because I've always wanted to visit Stockholm.

What we do know is that type 2 diabetes is increasing throughout the world at an alarming rate. It seems to be increasing the most in developing countries, especially when rural residents living a traditional lifestyle move to urban areas and adopt a more Western lifestyle. (When I refer to *Western* in this book, I mean modern industrialized North American or European. By *non-Western,* I mean indigenous people living a traditional non-industrialized lifestyle in any part of the world.) When this happens, in most cases they eat more food, including more fat and more highly refined carbohydrate (starchy and sugary) foods. They usually get a lot less exercise as they use automobiles or buses instead of walking wherever they go. They also often move from a close-knit village society with a lot of social support and emphasis on the common good to an unfamiliar city where familiar social support is lacking and individuals are left to sink or swim on their own. In other words, their stress levels are increased.

No one is certain which of these factors is the most likely to cause type 2 diabetes. Is it the increase in total calories? The increase in fat consumption? The increase in refined carbohydrate consumption? The increase in stress? The decrease in exercise? Or a combination of several or all of these factors?

When people increase their total food intake and reduce their activity level, they usually gain weight. Thus the increase in diabetes rates usually goes along with an increase in obesity. Some people thus think that obesity causes diabetes. However, as I'll explain later, the situation is more complicated than that. Not everyone who becomes overweight gets diabetes.

Nevertheless, activities that reduce weight—meaning eating less and exercising more—can also reduce the incidence of diabetes. Studies in several countries—including the United States, China, New Zealand, Sweden, and Finland—have proved this. In the U.S. Diabetes Prevention Program, more than three thousand people who were at high risk of diabetes were followed for almost three years. The group in which people lost about 7 percent of their weight and exercised (most chose walking) just thirty minutes a day for five days a week had 58 percent less diabetes than the control group.

Note that *reducing the risk* is not the same as *preventing*. Despite eating less and exercising more, some of the people in the studies still got diabetes. Some of the people who didn't get diabetes during the studies might get diabetes in five years or twenty years or forty years. Nevertheless, even postponing diabetes is beneficial, because the longer you have diabetes the more apt you are to have painful complications from the disease. If the preventive efforts had begun earlier and been more intense, it is possible that more people might have been able to avoid getting diabetes at least for many more years.

Both genes and environment are important

TYPE 2 DIABETES seems to be caused by an interaction of your genes and your environment. I say *seems to* because as I noted before, no one is entirely certain what causes type 2 diabetes. But here's how it's thought to work.

In order to get type 2 diabetes, you need "diabetes genes." If you don't have those genes, no matter what you do, how little you exercise, and how much you eat, you won't get diabetes, even if you get very fat. Conversely, if you have diabetes genes, you may not get the disease under certain conditions. In order to get type 2 diabetes, you need *both* the genes and a suitable environment to bring out those genes.

Let me explain by an analogy. Imagine (and this is obviously an imaginary example) that your family carried genes that made people produce little blue tufts of hair in the middle of their heads when they ate kangeroo meat. If your ancestors lived in Europe and didn't feel like importing a lot of kangaroo meat from Australia, they would never have sprouted blue tufts and would never have known that they carried the "blue tuft" genes. Conversely, Australians who didn't have the blue tuft genes could eat all the kangaroo meat they wanted and never get blue tufts.

But if you moved to Australia and started eating kangaroo meat, you would get blue tufts on your head. You might think, "It can't be genetic. No one in my family ever had blue tufts." But in fact, your family always had the genes. They just weren't in an environment that caused the genes to be expressed.

In order to get the blue tufts, you would need *both* the genes and the kangaroo meat. Type 2 diabetes is thought to be the same. But in this case the trigger that brings out the genes may be simply *too much food for the amount of physical work that you do.*

Some people think that type 2 diabetes genes are "thrifty genes" that allow a person to store fat very easily. This would come in very handy when you lived in an environment in which food was scarce, or when there were alternating good times and famine times. During the good times your body would store a lot of fat, and during the famine times you could live off the fat you had stored.

Unfortunately, the same genes may be a liability when you live in an enviroment in which food is plentiful, especially when it's high in calories and tasty and tempting. It's even more of a disaster when serving sizes in the society you live in are much larger than they need to be.

When thrifty genes and too much food occur in a person living in a society in which most people have machines to do the work and when they get from place to place in automobiles instead of walking or riding bicycles, you have a recipe for gaining a lot of weight. And, unfortunately, type 2 diabetes often goes along with the gain in weight.

The important thing about the thrifty genes is to understand that if you have these genes, you may need to work a lot harder than other people to keep obesity and type 2 diabetes at bay. It's not really fair. You surely know people who can eat all the fast food they want and drink soft drinks all day and snarf down candy bars whenever they pass a vending machine, but they're skinny as pencils, and they don't get diabetes.

In other words, if you eat the same things as your friends but put on a lot of weight when they don't, it may not be your fault. It's just that you have those thrifty genes. On the other hand, it's not wise to say, "Oh well. It's genetic. Nothing I can do about it." Remember, in order to get type 2 diabetes you need *both* the genes *and* the environment. You can't change your genes, but you *can* change your environment. It may require a lot of work and self-control, a lot more discipline than some other people need to have. But you *can* do it. You *can* make a difference to your health.

The basic prescription for a person with thrifty genes is simple: Eat less and move more. Well, it's simple to say. It's a lot more difficult to follow. In this book I will give you some suggestions for how you can put this simple mantra into action.

But now you may wonder, "How do I know if I have thrifty diabetes genes?" If your grandparents or your parents or your cousins or your siblings developed type 2 diabetes, you know the genes are in your family, and there's a chance that you have inherited them too. If you've always had a problem with easy weight gain, it's even more likely.

Certain ethnic groups are more apt to have thrifty genes than others. These include people in many different parts of the world: Native Americans, African Americans, Hispanics/Latinos, Pacific Islanders, Asians, Australian aboriginals, and peninsular Arabs. In fact, it has been suggested that the real minority here is people of European descent, who have type 2 diabetes rates of only about 6 percent, compared with rates close to 50 percent in some Native American and Pacific Island populations. If you have an ethnic background that puts you in one of the high-risk groups, you should be especially vigilant and try hard to reduce your risk factors.

Low birth weights have also been associated with higher rates of type 2 diabetes, so a child born during a famine in India who later moved to a city and got a good job and ate plentiful Western food would be even more likely to get type 2 diabetes. A possible illustration of this is a diabetes trend among Somali immigrants in Minnesota. Some of them are becoming diabetic within six months of adopting an American lifestyle—with weight gains of only ten or twenty pounds. In Somalia—where type 2 diabetes was practically unknown—they walked or rode bicycles to get from here to there, and food was not abundant or highly processed. In recent years, malnutrition has been one of the major medical problems in war-torn Somalia. Now the immigrants have both the labor-saving devices of modern American lifestyles and plenty to eat, perhaps for the first time in their lives.

Having gestational diabetes—a type of diabetes that occurs during the last few months of pregnancy and then usually goes away after the baby is born—is also a red flag for eventually getting type 2 diabetes. About 60 to 70 percent of people who have had gestational diabetes eventually are diagnosed with diabetes. Another red flag is central obesity, meaning a lot of fat in your stomach (often called the "apple shape") as opposed to weight in your thighs and butt ("pear shape").

Excess weight can cause insulin resistance

A LOT OF things about type 2 diabetes seem to come in pairs. In order to get the disease, you need to have both the genes and a food-rich, exercise-poor environment. Here's another thing that involves a pair. Most people with type 2 diabetes have both *insulin resistance*, which I've already described, and a defect in the *beta cells* in the pancreas. What are beta cells? Well, insulin is produced in an organ behind the stomach called the *pancreas*. You've probably heard of that. When you eat the pancreas of an animal, it's called sweetbreads. The specialized cells in the pancreas that produce insulin are called *beta cells*.

The defect in the beta cells is mostly genetic, although the beta cells can also be damaged in an accident or by certain drugs and other chemicals. If a person without such a defect becomes insulin resistant—meaning they're producing insulin but the insulin isn't working very well—the beta cells can just keep cranking out more and more insulin to overcome the insulin resistance. It's as if the prices at the grocery store went up so your money was less effective. A rich person could keep getting more and more money from the bank to cope with the higher prices. A poor person couldn't.

Having a genetic defect in the beta cells is like having a low income. When the demand becomes greater, you can't cope with the higher needs. So a person with diabetic genes needs to do whatever is possible to keep those needs as low as possible.

One way to do this is to keep the insulin resistance down. Insulin resistance is partly genetic, and there's nothing you can do about that. But insulin resistance is also usually increased when you gain weight. And this is something you *can* try to control. Sometimes, losing weight will reduce your insulin resistance just enough so that your low-output beta cells can cover the lower needs and your blood glucose levels will remain in the normal range—one hopes forever.

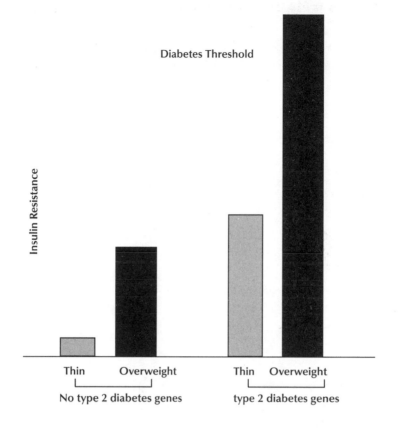

Figure 1. Insulin resistance and diabetes. Type 2 diabetes is thought to be caused by a combination of insulin resistance that you inherit plus insulin resistance that you acquire by gaining too much weight. In other words, both your genes and your lifestyle may play a role. See text for details.

Figure 1 shows how this works. The dotted line shows the level of insulin resistance that would cause diabetes. (The real situation is a little more complicated, as shown in Figure 2. But I've simplified it here. Once you understand the simple situation, the more complicated situation should be clearer.) Your genes determine how much genetic insulin resistance you have. You can see that a thin person without diabetes genes has very little insulin resistance. A thin person with diabetes genes has some insulin resistance, but it's not enough to go over the "diabetes threshold."

Now what happens when both those people gain weight? The person without diabetes genes acquires insulin resistance, but it's not enough to go over the diabetes threshold. It's only when you've got both diabetes insulin resistance genes *and* you become overweight that your insulin resistance sends you into the diabetic range.

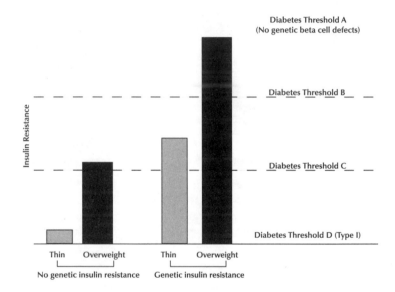

Figure 2. Beta cell defects and diabetes. In addition to insulin resistance, the amount of insulin that the beta cells in your pancreas can produce makes a difference in how likely you are to acquire type 2 diabetes. If your beta cells can produce a lot of insulin, you can have a lot of insulin resistance and still not get diabetes. If your beta cells can't produce much insulin, you can get type 2 diabetes even when you're not overweight. See text for details.

Even if you've gone over this level and you've been diagnosed with diabetes, *if you are diagnosed at an early stage,* sometimes losing weight will bring you back down below the diabetes threshold and your blood glucose levels will return to normal.

Figure 2 shows how differences in the capacity of your beta cells can determine how much insulin resistance you need to have to get diabetes. In this case, the graph shows four *different* thresholds, which depend on how much insulin your beta cells are able to produce.

At the top, Threshold A shows what happens in people who have no defects in their beta cells. Even if they had genetic insulin resistance and became hugely obese, they still wouldn't get diabetes, because their beta cells would just keep churning out enough insulin to cover the huge needs from the insulin resistance.

The next line down, Threshold B, shows the most common kind of type 2 diabetes, in which the beta cell threshold is high enough that it takes a combination of genetic insulin resistance *and* being overweight to go over the diabetes threshold, as shown in Figure 1.

The next line down, Threshold C, represents a person whose beta cells are able to produce enough insulin so that insulin shots are not needed. However, the beta cells produce a lot less insulin than normal. And if such a person also has insulin resistance, either because of insulin resistance genes *or* because of gaining a lot of weight, that person may develop type 2 diabetes. If the insulin resistance stems only from weight gain, that person may be able to reverse the condition by weight loss. If the insulin resistance is genetic, weight loss will have very little, if any, effect. Approximately 20 percent of people who develop type 2 diabetes are *not* overweight when they are diagnosed and may just have a very low beta cell output and hence a low diabetes threshold.

At the bottom, Threshold D, is a person whose beta cells produce almost no insulin at all. This would be typical of a person with type 1 diabetes. You can see that in this case, the amount of insulin resistance wouldn't matter. Even a thin person without genetic insulin resistance would become diabetic.

You can see that type 2 diabetes is very complicated. Different people have different degrees of insulin resistance and different degrees of insulin production by the beta cells. Thus depending on your genetic background, you could develop diabetes with different amounts of weight gain or different amounts of exercise—or its lack.

Diabetes can have serious complications

UNTREATED, DIABETES CAN lead to serious, sometimes fatal, complications, including blindness, amputations, kidney failure, and heart disease. If diagnosed early and controlled—which involves a lot of effort—the complications can usually be kept at bay for many years, sometimes forever.

But the best way to avoid diabetic complications is to avoid the disease altogether. As I've said, you can't control your genes. But you *can* reduce your risk factors by making sure you don't eat more than you need for your own particular activity level. If you choose not to move at all except between the couch and the refrigerator, then you'll need hardly any food at all. If you're a gymnast or if you're cutting down trees with an ax and then sawing them up with a handsaw, you'll need a lot more food. But even gymnasts and woodsmen can gain weight if the food they eat is excessively rich and abundant.

Take one step at a time

TOTALLY CHANGING YOUR lifestyle is difficult, and few people who aren't already diagnosed with diabetes have the motivation to do that. In fact, doing a complete lifestyle makeover overnight might not be a good idea. If you suddenly embark on a new lifestyle that includes a spartan diet of celery sticks, boiled skinless chicken, and skim milk, no smoking, no alcohol, no caffeine, and a five-mile run every day, you'll reduce your risk of getting diabetes. But you'll probably also increase your risk of burnout. If the program is *too* rigorous, you're apt to just give up and return to your former way of life.

Slowly making a lot of little changes that don't totally disrupt your life may have more effect in the long run, because you're more apt to stick with them. This book presents fifty different suggestions for things you can do to reduce your risk. If you try following one of the suggestions every week, by the end of a year you will have implemented them all—with a three-week vacation, because the first tip really encompasses all the rest—and greatly increased the chances that you won't develop type 2 diabetes for many years, if ever.

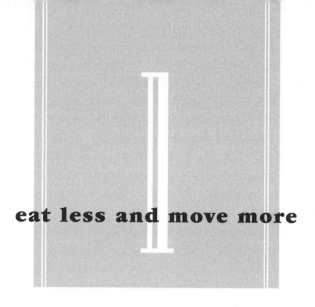

eat less and move more

Type 2 diabetes rates increase when people change their
lifestyle so that they eat more food and exercise less.

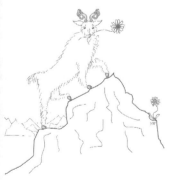

this first suggestion is
really the Mother of All Tips, and if it were
easy to implement, I wouldn't need to
write this book. "Eat less and move more"
is easy to say, but it's difficult to do.

I'm starting with it not because I expect
a lot of recliner potatoes will suddenly
think, "Oh. So that's it," throw away all the
rich foods in the house, start living off Swiss chard and broccoli
sprouts, train for the New York marathon, and solve all their
problems.

I'm starting with it because it *is* the philosophy underlying
all the following tips, and it's easy to remember. If you're ever

facing a new lifestyle decision and you want to know how it would affect your diabetes risk, just ask yourself, "Would this help me to eat less and move more?" and take the answer into consideration when making your decision.

For example, let's say you're thinking of moving to a new apartment and you have two different possibilities, both the same price. Apartment A is right next to the subway and a block away from a fast-food takeout restaurant, so it would be very convenient to pick up some supper on your way home from your exhausting job. Apartment B is six blocks from the subway and two blocks from a health food store that sells reasonably priced fresh produce. Apartment A sounds a lot more convenient, but if you got Apartment B, you'd get more exercise walking to the subway every day, and you'd be more apt to eat healthier foods if they were nearby.

Notice that I don't say, "Exercise more." The important factor in preventing diabetes is to let your muscles work, but not necessarily in formal exercises. Visualize Native American societies before Europeans arrived on the continent. Did they spend a lot of time at aerobics classes or walking on stair-stepping machines? Of course not. They also had almost no type 2 diabetes. But they didn't suffer from an overabundance of rich food, and simply carrying out the tasks of daily life gave their bodies a good workout.

Your goal should be to come as close as feasible to that way of life. Try to work moving your muscles into your daily routine rather than limiting exertion as much as possible all day and then spending time at an exercise club. Park as far from where you're going as possible. Take the stairs instead of the elevator. Walk to a nearby store instead of driving. Move your mailbox a little farther from the house. Walk to a neighborhood store for your newspaper every day instead of having it delivered.

eat less and move more

Eat only what you need—with occasional breaks for celebrations. Note that in people already diagnosed with diabetes, it has been shown that blood glucose control improves when people start eating less *even before they have lost any weight.* Presumably, the same would be true for those who are not yet diabetic. So even if you're one of those people who seems to gain weight on a diet of steamed grass and water, eating less should reduce the chances that your blood sugar level will reach diabetic levels.

If you find weight loss extremely difficult and just can't seem to lose weight no matter what you do, don't despair. Focus on getting more exercise. Studies have shown that overweight people who are physically fit are actually healthier than skinny couch potatoes. One study showed that people who exercise reduce their risk of getting diabetes just as much as those who diet as well as exercising more.

Here's another benefit from eating less food: Studies in animals have shown that when you limit their food, they live significantly longer than animals allowed to eat as much as they want. So if you eat less, not only are you going to look better, feel better, and reduce your chances of getting diabetes, but you're also going to have a longer life in which to enjoy all these benefits.

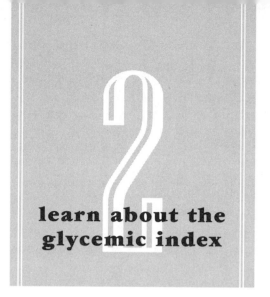

learn about the glycemic index

R A T I O N A L E :

Low–glycemic index foods are digested more slowly and don't raise blood glucose levels as fast as high–glycemic index foods. A high intake of high–glycemic index foods has been associated with an increased risk of type 2 diabetes.

the food you eat consists of proteins (for example, meat, fish, and eggs), fats (butter and oils), and carbohydrates (sugars, and starches such as flour, potatoes, and rice). Carbohydrate foods have the greatest impact on your blood glucose levels because most carbohydrates that are digested by the body consist of long chains of glucose molecules. As you digest your food, the carbohydrates are broken down into glucose.

Not all carbohydrate foods raise blood glucose levels at the same rate, however. Scientists have tested a lot of carbohydrate foods and classified them according to how quickly a certain amount of carbohydrate in a food makes blood glucose levels go up compared with white bread or glucose.

Then they gave each food a number to indicate the food's ability to increase blood glucose levels. This number is called the *glycemic index* of the food.

Table 1 shows some glycemic index values. You may be surprised by some of the results. Rice cakes and potatoes raise blood glucose levels faster than table sugar (sucrose) and candy (chocolate bar). Note also that the type of a particular food can make a difference. White-skinned, peeled, boiled potatoes have a lower glycemic index than mashed red-skinned potatoes. Different varieties of rice can have different glycemic index values. Foods with high glycemic index values are sometimes called *fast carbohydrates.*

You may wonder what this has to do with preventing diabetes. Probably a lot. When you don't have diabetes, eating some fast carbohydrates shouldn't hurt you. The beta cells in your pancreas also work fast and just churn out a lot of insulin, which keeps the blood glucose level in the normal range. But if you eat tremendous amounts of such foods, you are flooding your bloodstream with a lot of glucose at once. If you have diabetes genes and your pancreas isn't able to produce huge amounts of insulin—and especially if you have insulin resistance as well—your pancreas may not be able to cope, and your blood glucose level will go up.

High blood glucose levels, in turn, are toxic to the beta cells, causing further damage, which limits their ability to produce insulin even more. In other words, you're caught in a vicious circle.

Lower-glycemic foods are digested more slowly, releasing into your bloodstream a slow trickle of glucose that is less stressful for your beta cells.

The glycemic index applies only to carbohydrate foods. Proteins and fats raise the blood glucose level so little that researchers haven't focused on measuring the glycemic index of foods that are mainly fat or protein. Also, the glycemic index tells you only how much a particular food will raise your blood glucose levels compared with another food if you eat the same amount (researchers used fifty grams) of digestible carbohydrate in each food. Some foods like potatoes contain mostly starch, which is a quickly digestible carbohydrate. Some foods like carrots have a high glycemic index but contain so little digestible carbohydrate that you'd have to eat an awful lot of carrots to get fifty grams of digestible carbohydrate.

Hence a newer concept called the *glycemic load* has been developed. The glycemic load is simply the glycemic index corrected for the amoun*t* of digestible carbohydrate in a food. Thus carrots, which have a high glycemic index, have a very small glycemic load. Lists of glycemic loads are currently available at *http://www.mendosa.com/gilists.htm* and appear in *The New Glucose Revolution*, being published in early 2003.

Because low-glycemic foods are often rich in indigestible fiber (see Tip 4), eating low–glycemic index foods also helps to fill you up without a lot of calories and often results in weight loss as well as protecting your beta cells.

The book *The Glucose Revolution* contains the most complete list of glycemic index values. If you have access to the Internet, search on "glycemic index" and you should find Rick Mendosa's glycemic index page (currently at *www.mendosa.com/gi.htm*) as well as a searchable database run by the Australian researchers who helped develop the concept (currently at *http://www.glycemicindex.com/*).

In non-Westernized societies that have low diabetes rates, the carbohydrate foods people eat are usually close to their native state. They may be cooked or pounded or ground with stones, but they aren't highly refined as many of the carbohydrates we eat are—for example, white flour. Refining foods usually increases their glycemic index because it breaks the coarse carbohydrate foods down into extremely fine particles that are digested very quickly (see Figure 4 with Tip 8).

Thus one reason for low diabetes rates in non-Westernized societies may be that the carbohydrates they eat have low glycemic index values. Studies of Americans have shown that increased consumption of foods with low glycemic index values, such as whole grains, reduces the incidence of diabetes in both men and women.

Cooking also increases the glycemic index because it makes the carbohydrates more accessible to the digestive enzymes. Thus spaghetti that is barely cooked—al dente—has a lower glycemic index than overcooked or canned spaghetti. Stewed vegetables have higher glycemic index values than quickly stir-fried vegetables.

Raw foods have the lowest glycemic index values of all. In most cases, however, it's not realistic to expect you to convert to a raw-food diet. Furthermore, some foods are not particularly healthy when eaten raw. Moderation is the key here. Try to eat more fresh, uncooked foods like raw carrots and salads, and try not to overcook your stews and soups.

Stress lightly cooked, low–glycemic index foods, but don't totally deprive yourself of all the well-cooked foods you enjoy. It's important to enjoy life as well as to be aware of the glycemic index values of the foods you eat. Focus on the low–glycemic index foods for everyday fare and save the others for special occasions.

TABLE 1

GLYCEMIC INDEX VALUES OF SOME COMMON FOODS

Tofu frozen dessert, low fat	115
Parsnips, boiled	97
French baguette	95
Potato, red-skinned, mashed	91
Rice cakes	82
Cheerios, General Mills	74
Bagel	72
White bread	70
Cornmeal	68
Sucrose	65
Potato, new, unpeeled, boiled	62
Banana	55
Frosted Flakes, Kellogg's	55
Whole-grain pumpernickel bread	51
Chocolate bar	49
Oatmeal, old-fashioned	49
Grapefruit juice	48
Macaroni	45
Orange, navel	44
Apple	38
Black beans, boiled	30
Milk	27
Barley, pearled	25
Grapefruit	25
Yogurt, plain	14

These values, taken from data in the book *The Glucose Revolution* (1st edition, Marlowe 1999), represent glycemic index values relative to glucose, which has a glycemic index of 100.

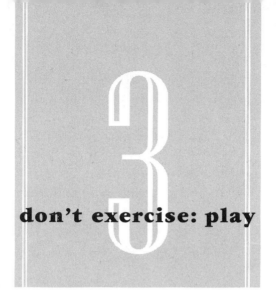

don't exercise: play

Moving as much as possible exercises your muscles
and helps to reduce your diabetes risks. But there's
no reason that moving more has to be a bore.

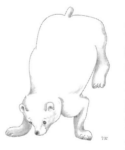

if you enjoy working out at a
gym, jogging down a road, or doing push-
ups on the living room floor, that's great.
Keep it up. The exercise will do a lot to
keep type 2 diabetes at bay. This is
because exercise improves the ability of
your muscles to remove glucose from the
blood: it decreases your insulin resistance. There is also evidence that exercise increases the amount of fat you burn for
energy instead of storing it in your fat cells.

But for many of us, formal exercises are a bore. For some,
they may be a reminder of high school gym classes with Mr.
Moveyerbutt, who had you doing tedious calisthenics in a
smelly gym when you would much have preferred to be outside playing soccer or baseball.

If you're still in school, the opportunities to join a sport should be available. If your school has teams only for the gifted athletes and you're always on the bench, lobby for some kind of activity that would work for you. You're undoubtedly not the only one in that situation.

If you're older, your age doesn't mean you have to stop playing. The trick is to find some kind of "play" that is convenient, affordable, and possible. If you like moving to music, an aerobics class may fill the bill. If not, are there any group sports in your neighborhood? An adult soccer team? Baseball? Why don't you organize a team?

Do you like to swim? Have you ever tried snowshoeing or cross-country skiing? Have you always wanted to try hitting a tennis ball? Why not try now?

If even thinking of such strenuous play tires you out, then start with something a little less rigorous. Walk. Don't just walk on a treadmill or up and down the same road day after day. That's too much like exercise. Instead, turn your walk into play. If you enjoy company, persuade some friends to go along and have a nice chat as you go.

Explore new areas of your city or your suburb or your rural environment. Learn about the architecture of your town or the habits of wild critters in your neighborhood, and seek out new adventures every time you walk.

If you live in an area of the city that isn't safe for walking, consider taking the bus or subway to another area of town where it is safe. Go to a mall and walk there. Or find a free museum and walk around there. The benefit to your health should outweigh the cost of the bus fare. Take some friends along and make it an outing to look forward to several times a week. Or organize a walking club, so there will be safety in numbers.

When moving more means having more fun, you'll be more apt to stick with it and fight off those diabetes genes.

don't exercise: play

4

learn to fill up on high-fiber foods

RATIONALE:

No one likes to feel hungry. High-fiber carbohydrate foods fill your stomach without many calories and reduce your hunger for many hours after you eat them.

digestible carbohydrates have the greatest effect on your blood sugar levels. But not all carbohydrates are digestible. Carbohydrates come in several different types. The simplest are the sugars, whose names usually end in *-ose*, for example, glucose (blood sugar), sucrose (table sugar), and lactose (milk sugar). Another type of carbohydrate is starch, which I discuss in detail in Tip 13. Both sugars and starches are quickly digested and raise your blood glucose levels quite fast.

But there's another type of carbohydrate that our bodies can't digest very well, or not at all. This is *fiber*. Our grandparents called it *roughage* and emphasized its importance in maintaining "regularity," meaning regular, painless bowel movements.

Fiber consists of carbohydrates that human enzymes can't digest—for example, cellulose, an exception to the rule that words ending in -*ose* are sugars. Because humans can't digest carbohydrates like cellulose, they are calorie-free, as far as we're concerned, and pass right through us.

However, fibers also have a lot of bulk. Think of eating a bale of hay. You wouldn't get a lot of nutrition from the hay, except for a few dried bugs that might be in the bale. But it sure would fill you up. And because hunger pangs can be satisfied by a full stomach as well as by an increase in the blood sugar level, high-fiber foods can do a lot to make you feel full without adding to your calorie intake.

Fiber has other benefits as well. I've already mentioned the effects of fiber on "regularity." That's mostly an effect of what is called *insoluble fiber* because it is (big surprise) insoluble in water. Think of sawdust, which is an insoluble cellulose fiber. Foods high in insoluble fiber include bran cereals, whole grains, beans, and plant stems, leaves, and skin, that is, the "tough" parts of fruits and vegetables.

There's another kind of fiber called *soluble fiber* because (and I'll bet you can guess the answer here) it is soluble in water. Soluble fibers form gooey gels, like jelly or gelatin dessert. Okra has a lot of soluble fiber, as do oatmeal, nopal cactus, and aloe vera. Other sources of soluble fiber are fruits, beans, cereal grains (oats, rice, barley), seed contents, and seaweed, that is, the "succulent" parts of fruits and vegetables. Thus if you eat whole fruits and vegetables, you're getting both insoluble and soluble fiber in one package.

Soluble fiber doesn't have a lot to do with regularity, but it has a lot to do with the speed at which you digest your food. The soluble fibers form gels in your stomach that make your stomach empty more slowly. The gels in your intestines protect some of the carbohydrates from the digestive enzymes, so the carbohydrates are digested much more slowly.

Both these effects mean that instead of presenting your

bloodstream with a sudden huge influx of glucose from a carbohydrate meal, an influx that your pancreas may have difficulty handling, the sugars in your meal are released more slowly, causing a slow and steady increase in blood sugar that even a wimpy pancreas may be able to deal with.

In their natural state, many carbohydrates are bound up with both soluble and insoluble fibers that both fill you up and give you a slow, steady release of glucose into the blood. In other words, high-fiber foods are usually low–glycemic index foods, which are associated with lower rates of diabetes. When these foods are highly processed, or refined, they are usually separated from the "useless" fibers, and these beneficial effects are lost. Their glycemic index increases.

If you're trying to reduce your calorie intake, it's a big help to seek high-fiber foods that will fill you up with their bulk, to reduce your hunger right away, as well as slowly releasing sugars over many hours, thus reducing your hunger for a long time as well.

Before I was diagnosed with diabetes, I occasionally ate a budget brand of TV dinners that had delicious sauces on pasta but very small portion sizes. That's one way manufacturers of such meals can advertise very few calories or a very low fat content: they simply don't give you much food. After eating one of those things, I didn't feel satisfied, although I liked the taste. So I learned to add French-style green beans. These added bulk with very few extra calories, soaked up the sauces, added something extra to chew, and made me feel full.

Here are a few more suggestions for substituting easty-to-eat high-fiber vegetables for starches:

❑ Use pureed cauliflower instead of mashed potatoes. Cook cauliflower until soft and puree in food processor with a little milk, cream, or cheese.
❑ Cut up raw cauliflower into rice-sized pieces. The easiest way to do this is to use a food processor. Put

into a glass bowl. Microwave for two or three minutes without extra liquid. Use instead of rice.
❑ Cut up and cook broccoli as above. Microwave a few minutes until bright green. Drizzle with olive oil and lemon juice. Serve decorated with red pepper slices and black olives.
❑ Lightly sauté onion and a mixture of summer squashes. Puree together.
❑ Substitute spaghetti squash for spaghetti. It has a different texture but makes a pleasant change and has very few calories.
❑ Substitute zucchini pancakes for potato pancakes.

Use your imagination to figure out more ways of making vegetables attractive and easy to eat.

An example of the benefits of a high-fiber carbohydrate is *tepary beans*, a special kind of bean that was grown and eaten by the Pima Indians in Arizona. Before a long march, during which there was no time to stop for a snack, the Pima made sure to eat tepary beans. It was said that you could work all day long on one meal of teparies. This is because instead of giving a sudden rush of sugar followed by hunger pangs, as sugary or starchy food would, the teparies were slow to digest and released nourishment slowly all day long.

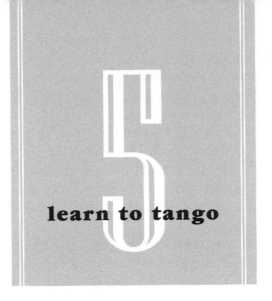

learn to tango

Your goal is to move more, and dancing is wonderful exercise. It can also be a lot of fun.

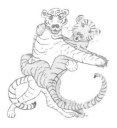

so ok, you don't need to tango if that's not a dance that appeals to you. Then how about learning to waltz? If you're young and waltzing seems as old-fashioned to you as the minuet, that might make it even more interesting. Try to persuade some of your friends to join you and get someone to teach you all.

If waltzing was standard fare at dancing school when you went, way back when, how long has it been since you and your partner stepped out to go dancing? No suitable dance spots in the neighborhood? No problem. Just put on a CD or a tape—even a record will do—and dance around the kitchen several times a week. It should be a lot more fun than working a stair stepper at the gym, and it's free. Make it even more special by getting dressed up in your fancy dancing duds and having a special dinner before your dancing evening.

Of course, it takes two to tango—and also to waltz. No partner? No problem. Why not learn some kind of solo dancing, like tap dancing. Think of Fred Astaire. I'll bet he never had to worry about getting diabetes. Just one of his routines must have burned off hundreds of calories and made his insulin resistance go way down. And he surely rehearsed many of them every day.

Square dancing is also excellent exercise, as is contra dancing. Some of these dances welcome beginners and teach you the beginning steps before the first dance. If not, try to enroll at a class in a local adult education program.

Various ethnic groups have their own forms of dance. Seek them out and see if you can learn. Try the hula. Get a group together and learn to minuet. Look into modern dance. Or just try whatever is hot with the young people today. Almost any kind of dancing will work out a lot of different muscles and provide social contacts as well.

If you're really adventuresome, take up belly dancing. Most of us with diabetes genes are very gifted in the belly area and should be the stars of the class even before the first lesson. If you're male, you'll have to be especially adventuresome to take up a traditional female dance. But why not? It burns calories.

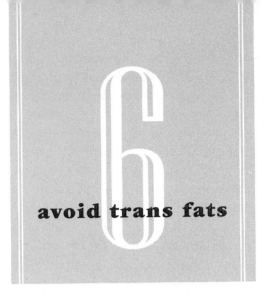

avoid trans fats

R A T I O N A L E :

Trans fats are unnatural manufactured fats that may have harmful effects on the body. A high intake of trans fats has been associated with an increased risk of type 2 diabetes.

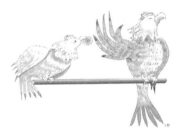

some fat in your diet is necessary. All the membranes of your cells contain fatty acids (which are the building blocks of fat). If you don't eat enough fat, your body will manufacture most of what you need. However, there are a few fats that your body is unable to make and must get from the diet. These include two fatty acids with the confusing names *linoleic acid* and *alpha-linolenic acid*. It's not necessary to remember the names of the essential fatty acids. What is important is to understand that not all fats are bad; you need some fats.

For the past several decades, Americans have been bombarded with messages telling us to "get the fat out" of our diets, and food manufacturers, eager to benefit from the public health campaign, have filled the shelves with manufactured low-fat and fat-free foods. As a result, many Americans have become so fat-phobic that the presence of even a little vegetable oil in a food may make them shun it. More recently, however, nutritionists and others have begun to publicize the fact that not all fats are bad. In fact, some fats seem to be beneficial. Thus it may be more important for you to focus on the *type* of fat you're eating rather than just the amount of fat in your diet.

To understand all this, it helps to understand just a little bit about the chemistry of fats. Like people, fats and oils (liquid fats) come in all shapes and sizes. All fats consist of long chains of carbon and hydrogen called *fatty acids* attached to a molecule of glycerin (which scientists call *glycerol*). Because there are usually three of the fatty acids attached to the glycerin molecule, the fats are sometimes called *triglycerides*.

Most of the carbon atoms in the fatty acids are "saturated" by all the hydrogen atoms that they can hold. Each carbon atom binds two hydrogen atoms. Fats made from fatty acids that are totally saturated are called, not surprisingly, *saturated fats*. Saturated fatty acids are long straight chains. Foods such as fatty red meat, dairy products, and tropical oils contain a lot of saturated fats.

But the carbon atoms in a fatty acid can also lose some of their hydrogen atoms and form what is called a *double bond* instead. When a fatty acid has a double bond it is called *unsaturated*. When it has only one such bond, it is called *monounsaturated*. Monounsaturated fatty acids are usually long chains with a kink somewhere along the chain. Foods such as olive oil, canola oil, nuts, and avocados contain a lot of monounsaturated fats.

When the fat has several unsaturated bonds, the fatty acid is called *polyunsaturated*. Polyunsaturated fats can be various shapes. Foods such as vegetable oils—for example, corn oil, safflower oil—contain a lot of polyunsaturated fats. Fats containing double bonds become oxidized very easily, and oxi-

avoid trans fats

dized fats are thought to contribute to heart disease. The popular word for oxidized fats is *rancid*. Polyunsaturated fats have more double bonds and are thus more easily oxidized than monounsaturated fats. Thus unless polyunsaturated oils are fresh or protected from rancidity by keeping them cold in dark bottles, or by adding antioxidants, they may be harmful.

Note that no one food contains only one type of fatty acid. Fats are usually classified according to the major type. Even red meat contains only about 50 percent saturated fat, and even olive oil contains some saturated fat.

The more unsaturated a fat is—the more double bonds it has—the more liquid it is at room temperature. This is why safflower oil, a highly unsaturated fat, is liquid, and we call it an oil. Butter, which contains mostly saturated fat, is solid at room temperature. Butter has always been more expensive than vegetable oils, and in the twentieth century, chemists learned how to use high temperatures and pressures to manufacture solid fats like vegetable shortening and margarine from cheap vegetable oils by forcing hydrogen atoms onto carbon atoms, replacing the double bonds.

At the time, it seemed like a wonderful idea. As long as the hydrogenation is complete, the result is simply saturated fats, which are found in nature. These are not a problem. But as time passed, it was discovered that when the process is not complete—when it produces *partially hydrogenated* fats— some of those fats assume an unnatural shape called a *trans fat*.

When people eat a standard American diet, including a lot of calories and a lot of carbohydrates as well as a lot of protein and fat, it has been shown that a high intake of saturated fat is associated with heart disease. Thus if you're eating a standard American diet, most nutritionists recommend trying to reduce the amount of saturated fat in your diet to lower your risks of heart disease. Furthermore, there is evidence that saturated fat increases insulin resistance, and insulin resistance increases your risks of getting diabetes.

Some people now think that trans fats are even more

unhealthy than saturated fats and may also affect your risk of getting diabetes. A recent report on a Harvard study of more than 80,000 nurses in the Boston area (called the Nurses Study) showed that although the total fat intake was unrelated to the incidence of diabetes, eating more trans fats caused diabetes rates to increase. On the other hand, eating more polyunsaturated fat (nontropical vegetable oil and fish oils) caused the diabetes rates to decrease. The authors estimated that simply replacing 2 percent of the trans fat in the diet by unsaturated fats could reduce the risk of type 2 diabetes by 40 percent or even more.

How do you know what foods have trans fats? Currently, most food labels (see Tip 17) don't mention the amount of trans fats in a product, but if you see the term *partially hydrogenated* in the list of ingredients, you can be certain the product contains trans fats. The trans fat content of stick margarines is usually high. Trans fats are also often found in baked goods and in crackers, cookies, and snack chips. These foods also usually have high glycemic index values. So by avoiding foods containing trans fats you will also be avoiding refined foods with high glycemic index values and hence reducing your risks of diabetes in two different ways at once.

SOURCES OF TRANS FAT

Breakfast cereals	French fries
Breakfast pastries	Frozen dinners
Cakes	Mayonnaise and salad dressing
Chips	Pies
Cookies	Stick margarine
Crackers	Vegetable shortening
Doughnuts	

These are the types of foods that may contain trans fats. Not all such products do contain trans fats. Check ingredients for terms like *partially hydrogenated, margarine,* and *vegetable shortening.*

avoid trans fats

listen to recorded books or music when your workout is routine

R A T I O N A L E :

When you want to keep active with a duller activity,
you can make the experience pleasurable if you
combine it with something you enjoy.

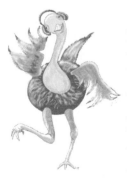

ideally, you'll be active doing things you enjoy, whether they be horseback riding, doing the tango, boxing, belly dancing, or just walking and chatting with good friends. But there are times when those activities aren't possible, for example, when it rains or when you're too busy to spend several hours preparing for and carrying out some enjoyable pastime.

If you want to continue to be active, you may sometimes turn to less stimulating forms of exercise, for example, walking on a treadmill, riding an exercise bicycle, lifting weights, stacking wood, or anything else routine enough that you don't have to pay a lot of attention as you do it.

Now, there are some people who get a thrill out of such activities, but I'm not one of them. If you can spend hours on an exercise bicycle and be happy as a clam (although I'm not sure exactly how a clam would pedal a bike), that's great. You're lucky. For me they are, well, dull. So I to listen to recorded books when I'm doing such activities. I get the tapes from the public library, usually several at a time to make sure at least one of them turns out to be really interesting. Then I don't let myself listen to the books except when I'm exercising.

When the book is really gripping, it means I actually look forward to an activity I don't particular enjoy—for example, lifting weights—because it means I get to hear more of the book. Tapes are also useful if you walk the same route every day—or walk on a treadmill—and get bored with the scenery.

Those little tape players that you can tie to your waist and listen to with earphones are great for this. You can buy one for about ten dollars at any drugstore or similar outlet. More and more books are becoming available on CDs, so you might want to look into a portable CD player instead.

I've heard dozens of great books this way, books I'd always wanted to read but didn't have time for. When a book is really engrossing, I find I don't even notice the hills when I'm walking. My mind is far away. If you're interested in self-education, you can also get tapes of college-course lectures, or learn a new language, or listen to a how-to tape as you get your muscles into shape.

Of course, if you'd rather listen to music, that would work just as well. Again, the trick is to have some special music you love and not to let yourself listen except when you're getting some exercise as well.

learn what processed, or refined, carbohydrates are— and don't overdose on them

R A T I O N A L E :

Highly refined carbohydrates usually have high glycemic index values, and a high intake of highly refined carbohydrates has been associated with an increased rate of type 2 diabetes.

in their natural state, most carbohydrate foods have low glycemic index values and are healthy. When they are highly refined (or processed—the words mean approximately the same thing), their glycemic index values usually go up.

Why is this? For several reasons. First, the refining process usually strips the starch from the fiber it was encased in. A good example is wheat. In its natural state, grains of wheat contain an outer hard coating, the *bran,* containing a lot of insoluble fiber; a starchy layer, which we turn into *flour*; and an inner vitamin-containing layer that we call *wheat germ.*

Unless the outer bran layer is somehow ruptured—by pounding, grinding, soaking and fermenting, or cooking—the grain of wheat is apt to pass right through you completely undigested. Figure 3 shows a fanciful view of three enzymes trying to get through the hard outer bran layer of some wheat so they can get to the starch. Even when the grains are partially cracked open—as in cracked wheat—whole grains are still in large chunks and have much of their starch attached to the bran layer, so it takes a long time for your digestive enzymes to process the starch. Hence digestion is slow.

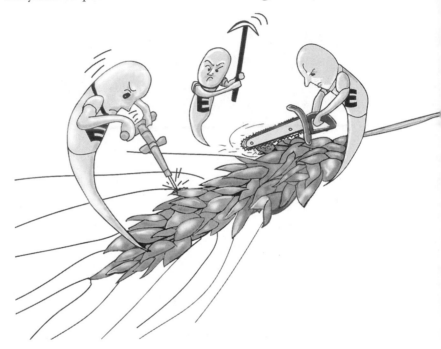

Figure 3. Digesting whole grains. This is a fanciful view of several enzymes trying to get through the tough bran layer on grains of wheat so they can reach the starch. They can't digest the starch in the wheat until the bran layer is breached by pounding, grinding, cooking, or soaking and fermenting.

Most processed foods aren't made with the whole grains of wheat. Instead, manufacturers strip off the bran, remove the germ, and mill the remaining starchy portion until it's very fine flour, which they then bleach to make it nice and white. As a result of all this refining, your digestive enzymes have no

learn what processed, or refined, carbohydrates are

trouble digesting the starch. Digestion is extremely rapid, and your blood sugar may shoot up after eating a meal that consists mostly of refined carbohydrate foods. Remember, high blood glucose levels can be toxic to your beta cells.

The size of a hunk of starch makes a big difference in how quickly it can be digested. Figure 4A shows an imaginative view of enzymes attacking a huge chunk of starch. Although more than one enzyme can attack the chunk at once, they only have access to the outer layer of the starch. The inner layers are digested only after the outer layers are removed. Thus although digestion is faster than it would be if the chunk was covered by a hard bran layer, it is still relatively slow. Figure 4B shows the same enzymes when the starch has been milled into fine bits. Now hundreds of enzymes can quickly "eat" (break down) the tiny bits of starch—just as you can quickly shovel a huge spoonful of rice into your mouth

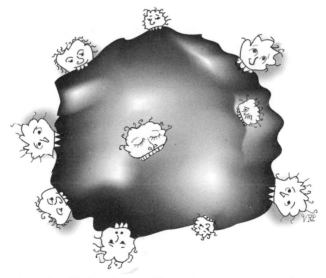

Figure 4. Coarsely milled grains are digested more slowly than finely milled grains. A. A fanciful view of some enzymes digesting a coarsely milled grain of starch. Although more than one enzyme can attack the grain at once, only the surface of the grain can be attacked. The bulk of the starch is in the interior of the grain. It can't be digested until the outer coats are slowly broken down. Hence digestion is relatively slow.

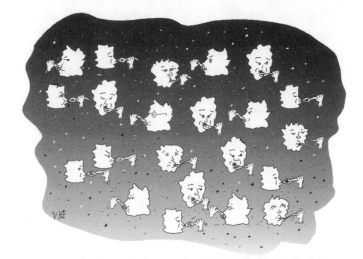

Figure 4. B. A fanciful view of some enzymes digesting finely milled grains of starch. Because the starch is now broken down into tiny bits, hundreds or thousands of enzymes can work on the starch at once. Hence digestion is rapid.

Farmers have to be aware of the differences between refined grains, cracked grains, and whole grains. If you feed a cow whole dried corn, much of the corn will pass right through it, and you'll have spent money on feed that was wasted. Cracked corn is more easily digested. However, if you mill the corn too finely, the cow will digest it too quickly, the stomach will become acidic, and the cow will get sick with "grain bloat." So farmers avoid highly milled grains for their animals. It's too bad we don't treat ourselves as well as we treat our farm animals.

Most "convenience foods" are high in refined carbohydrates, for example, crackers, white bread, breakfast cereals (except whole grains), cookies, and reconstituted potato chips or similar snacks. Even foods that are described as "healthy" because they are low in fat may contain huge amounts of refined carbohydrate in the form of wheat flour or cornstarch thickeners or large portions of well-cooked pasta.

learn what processed, or refined, carbohydrates are

Breakfast is a time when many Americans eat primarily highly processed carbohydrates. Except for whole-grain cereals such as old-fashioned oatmeal or a few high-bran cereals, most breakfast cereals are nothing but starch, sugar, and a little flavoring. Add to this a piece of white toast or bagel, jam, and orange juice, all foods with high glycemic index values, and you have a recipe for a rapid blood sugar rise followed several hours later by a crash.

Studies have shown that people who eat more refined carbohydrates have higher rates of type 2 diabetes. Many processed foods also contain trans fats (not to mention a lot of salt, which isn't directly related to your diabetes risk but is not good for your heart). So by avoiding refined foods as much as you can, you're avoiding two bad things at once.

If you ever become diabetic, you'll have to greatly limit your consumption of processed carbohydrates. You'll even have to keep track of all the carbohydrates you eat in more natural forms. This isn't a lot of fun.

You're much better off avoiding refined carbohydrates as much as you can *before* you become diabetic. That way, you can still occasionally splurge, and the damage won't be very great. As I said before, it's important to enjoy life. Don't think you have to give up refined carbohydrates completely. Just make sure they don't constitute the bulk of your diet.

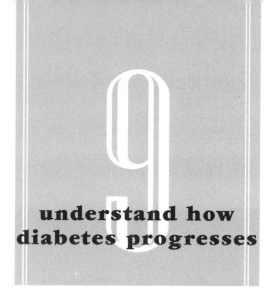

understand how diabetes progresses

R A T I O N A L E :

If you understand how diabetes progresses from normal blood glucose control to prediabetes to full-blown diabetes, you'll be better able to understand lab tests and stop the disease in the early stages.

type 2 diabetes doesn't just suddenly appear from nowhere like a bolt of lightning, even though it may feel that way if you're handed such a diagnosis. Instead, diabetes usually progresses slowly from normal blood glucose control through various intermediate stages until your control finally becomes so poor that you are diagnosed as diabetic. In fact, most people have had poor blood glucose control for ten or even twenty years before they are diagnosed, and they don't even know it.

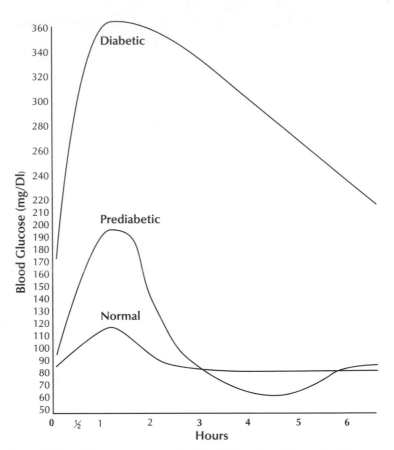

Blood Glucose (mg/Dl)

Hours

Figure 5. How diabetes progresses. The blood glucose level of people with no signs of diabetes (Normal) may go up to 120 mg/dL or even slightly higher (depending on the meal) after they eat. When you're beginning to lose control of your blood sugar levels (prediabetes), your blood glucose levels may be close to normal when you wake up in the morning and before meals. After meals, the levels go higher than normal. And about four hours after eating, they may drop lower than normal, causing symptoms of "low blood sugar." Once you're diabetic, even the fasting and premeal blood glucose levels will be above normal. You'll go even higher after meals, and it may take hours to return to the starting point.

Figure 5 shows how this works. The graph at the bottom shows what happens to blood glucose levels in a nondiabetic person after eating a normal meal, which was consumed at time zero. The blood glucose may go up to 120 milligrams per

understand how diabetes progresses

deciliter (mg/dL—the units used in the American system of measuring blood glucose levels) between one and two hours after the meal, and it then slowly falls back to the starting point, usually within a couple of hours, taking longer if the meal was a large one.

The next curve shows what happens in a person who is developing diabetes when the condition hasn't progressed very far. In this case, *note that the starting level is almost the same as that of the nondiabetic person,* well within the normal range (up to 126 mg/dL). However, after eating the same meal, this person sees a much higher rise in the blood glucose level, peaking at almost 200 mg/dL. Because the peak is higher, it also takes longer for it to come down.

Now look at what happens at about four or five hours after the meal: *the blood glucose level actually falls below normal* (blood sugar is considered low below about 50 to 70 mg/dL, depending on the individual and the method used to test the level). This is quite common in people who have early signs of becoming diabetic. About four or five hours after eating, you may notice signs of low blood sugar: shakiness, nervousness, and intense hunger, and you may have learned that eating something sweet stops these symptoms.

What this means is that your body is losing tight control of its blood glucose levels. Some people call it having a "sluggish pancreas." The beta cells don't produce enough insulin right after a meal to keep the blood glucose level down, and then when they start producing insulin, because the blood glucose level is so high by this time, they produce too much and your blood glucose levels go too low.

This condition used to be called *impaired glucose tolerance* (IGT), but in 2002 the name was changed to *prediabetes,* and diabetes specialists emphasized the need to diagnose people with this condition to reverse it before it progressed to full-blown diabetes. In the past, prediabetes was also sometime called "borderline diabetes," and sometimes doctors would just tell people their blood sugar was a bit high. It doesn't matter what you call it. The condition means you're at an extremely high risk of progressing to full-blown diabetes. Some people live with prediabetes for years before they're diagnosed with diabetes.

The top curve shows what might happen when a person with full-blown type 2 diabetes has a meal. Note that in this case, the starting point is well above normal. The blood glucose level then zooms to an extremely high level and, because it is so high, takes hours to approach its starting point. In fact, a person may already have begun a second meal before the high blood glucose level from the first meal has returned to the starting point.

One important thing to remember from this graph is that the premeal starting point for a nondiabetic person and a person with prediabetes may be very similar. The premeal blood glucose level is usually similar to what is called the *fasting level*, which means the blood glucose level that you have when you wake up in the morning, having fasted all night. Because a diagnosis of diabetes usually involves measuring your fasting level, a person with prediabetes is often told there is nothing wrong, "No diabetes diagnosis for you." Naturally, such a person is apt to be quite relieved and returns home and continues an imprudent lifestyle involving a lot of processed carbohydrates, too many trans fats, and not a lot of exercise until the condition progresses to full-blown type 2 diabetes.

This is very sad, because when it's diagnosed in the very early stages, type 2 diabetes is more easily reversed. Remember when I said that high blood glucose levels are toxic to beta cells. When you're at the stage of prediabetes, your beta cells may still have their full capacity to secrete insulin. They just can't quite cope with high insulin resistance.

Then your blood glucose levels slowly increase. They don't take quantum leaps from normal to prediabetes to diabetes but gradually become higher and higher. I've simply shown three theoretical situations to clarify the stages. If you ignore it for too long, the high blood glucose levels may kill off a lot of your beta cells, and if that happens, even if you do everything possible to reduce your insulin resistance, you'll never again be able to have normal control of your blood glucose levels when you eat a meal. You'll have to carefully control your diet for the rest of your life.

Deciding when you actually have diabetes is somewhat arbitrary and changes as official bodies make pronouncements about what levels are OK. Not too long ago, your fasting levels had to be 140 mg/dL before you were considered diabetic. Today the number is 126. In the future it may be even lower. Normal fasting blood glucose levels are considered to be between about 60 and 110. In the figure, I used a level of about 85 because it's somewhere in the middle.

What this means is, if you know you're at a very high risk of getting type 2 diabetes—if you have parents and siblings with the disease, if you have a serious weight problem, if you've had gestational diabetes, or if you've had trouble with low blood sugar after meals—don't accept a normal fasting blood glucose level as proof that you're not diabetic. Talk with your doctor and make sure the doctor does further tests—for example, measuring your blood glucose level after a meal or doing a special test called the *hemoglobin A1c* that measures your average blood glucose level over the past month or so.

Early detection is the key to avoiding irreversible, full-blown diabetes.

10

understand that diets are controversial

R A T I O N A L E :

If you understand that none of the experts can agree on what the best diet is, you'll be better able to find a way of eating that works for you.

people have been squabbling about the best diet—both for those seeking to lose weight and those with diabetes —for centuries. They still can't agree.

Thus you'll hear some "diet gurus" swear that the best way to lose weight is to avoid carbohydrate foods and concentrate on proteins and fats. Others tell you to avoid fats and concentrate on carbohydrates. There are diets that focus on the glycemic index and diets that tell you that you need an exact carbohydrate:protein:fat ratio of 40:30:30. There are liquid diets that come in cans, and there are one-food diets that try to bore your appetite to death. Still other diets just restrict total calories, sometimes combining calories and carbohydrates, or calories and fiber, or calories and fat and calling the combinations by names that they hope will disguise the fact that you're counting calories at all.

Most of the diet approaches work for most people at least to some extent as long as you follow them strictly. The calorie-restricted approaches obviously work by restricting the number of calories you take in. Low-glycemic index diets work by filling you up with a lot of fiber, so you don't eat a lot of more fattening foods or high-glycemic carbohydrates. Low-fat diets work because fat has nine calories per gram and carbohydrate has only four calories per gram. By limiting the more calorie-dense foods, you may eat fewer calories without actually counting calories. Low-carbohydrate diets tend to work by dulling your appetite.

When something works for everyone, there's only usually one or two different varieties of the successful invention. For example, most cars use gasoline engines because gasoline engines work. But when you find dozens or even hundreds of different methods of trying to do one thing—in this case, help you lose weight—there's a good chance that none of them is 100 percent successful.

In fact there's some evidence that in general, any kind of diet will work for a short period of time, when it's all new and your enthusiasm is high. But people tend to get tired of any kind of restrictive way of eating, gradually revert to their former ways, and quickly regain all the weight they had lost—often even more. Some studies show that the only people who are successful at keeping their weight off long term are those who maintain an exercise program as well as the new way of eating prescribed by the diet.

Some people feel that any kind of diet is futile, that everyone has a *set point* that determines how much that person will weigh. Dieting to get below that set point simply triggers intense hunger and makes your metabolism go down, eventually making you regain all the lost weight. Even people in the well-publicized Diabetes Prevention Program seemed to have this problem despite intensive lifestyle support from a batallion of professionals. The average weight loss at six months was about fifteen pounds. By four years, the average weight loss had been reduced to only about nine pounds. People with "thrifty" diabetes genes often put on weight extremely easily and find it next to impossible to get that weight off again.

I know this all sounds pretty hopeless. But it's not. If you have a problem with weight, you have to accept that you're going to have to work harder on weight control than many other people for the rest of your life. Instead of going on a diet, reaching your goal, and then going back to "normal eating" because you're thin, you're going to have to eat modestly forever. It's not fair. But it's not fair that some people die from cancer when they're children and other people live to be 103.

Thus you have to find a diet—or a way of eating—that works for you and that you can live with for the rest of your life. Don't worry about what works for your friends. We all have slightly different metabolisms, and what is best for someone else may not be best for you.

Here's something to keep in mind: If you can find a way of eating that is able to control your weight now, *before* you get diabetes, then you'll occasionally be able to splurge and eat "forbidden" meals without causing great harm. If you wait until someone gives you a diabetes diagnosis, then your diet will have to be much, much stricter, and every time you waver from the straight and narrow path, you'll be increasing the chances that you'll develop diabetes complications.

Before you settle on a permanent way of eating, you might want to try several different approaches. It's unlikely you'll want to spend the rest of your life drinking meals out of cans or going to group meetings for weekly weigh-ins, and it wouldn't be healthy to spend the rest of your life on a real fad diet that didn't allow you to eat anything but carrot peels and grapefruit juice.

Some of these approaches may work fine for short-term weight loss, but you're looking for something long term, something that will help you keep the weight off rather than just letting you fit into smaller blue jeans for your high school reunion.

Look for a way of eating that lets you

- ❏ Eat the kinds of foods that you enjoy. If you love spaghetti and bread but aren't that keen on butter and fat, a low-fat diet would be a good choice. If you can't live without sour cream and steak but you think you can live without bread and rice, then a low-carb diet would be a better choice. If you can't imagine giving up any kind of food, then a portion-control or calorie-control diet would be a good place to start.
- ❏ Eat the kinds of foods that you can afford. If you're rich, there are no limits. But if you have a very limited budget, a low-carb diet, with its emphasis on meats and vegetables and ban on cheap starches, might be too expensive to be practical.
- ❏ Eat the kinds of food that are reasonably convenient for your lifestyle. If you work in an office or are going to school where the cafeteria offerings are limited, make sure either that you'll have time to pack a lunch to bring with you to work or that the foods on the diet you choose will be available there.

If you can afford it, a dietician can work with you to find out what approach to eating would be most suitable for you. If you decide to consult a dietician, make sure ahead of time that the person is open-minded and won't simply push you into the currently popular one-size-fits-all U.S. Department of Agriculture Food Pyramid diet. That diet *does* work for some people. Others—especially those with the kind of carbohydrate sensitivity that may go along with diabetes genes—find that they are constantly hungry on such a plan.

Remember that official bodies keep changing their pronouncements about healthy eating as new evidence comes in. Some years ago, everyone was supposed to stop using butter and olive oil and use margarine and safflower oil instead. Now some people say that margarine has too many trans fats and safflower oil becomes rancid too quickly to be healthy, and olive oil and even butter may be healthier after all. What's touted as "healthy" today may turn out to be "toxic" tomorrow. Use common sense, and don't go overboard with any one food, no matter how healthy today's experts say it is.

Get several books on weight-loss plans from the library or browse some in a bookstore, and see which ones make the most sense for you. Avoid diets that promise weight loss without any effort or huge losses in very short periods of time. They're always failures in the long run, and some of them are actually dangerous. Controlling your weight for the rest of your life is not an easy task. It's too bad they don't give Olympic medals for the people who are able to do it, because it requires enormous effort and dedication to succeed.

You may think, Why bother? Well, having diabetes is not a lot of fun, and dealing with it requires much more than just sticking to a spartan way of eating. Making the extra effort for the next twenty years may spare you from twenty years of having diabetes, and the longer you have diabetes, the greater the chance that you will suffer from complications.

So do some investigating. Learn a little about nutrition. And find a way of eating that will satisfy both your hunger and your tendency to gain weight, one that you can stick with for many years.

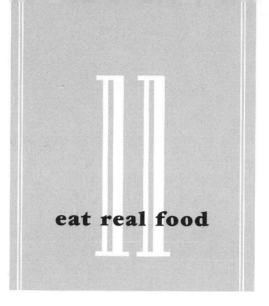

eat real food

R A T I O N A L E :

Non-Westernized people who eat foods close to their
natural state tend not to develop diabetes.

worldwide, the story is repeating itself. A
group of people—ranging from the Pima Indians in Arizona
to the Tiwi of Australia to the people of New Guinea to those
on the Pacific islands of Nauru and Tonga—have been living
for centuries off the fruits of the land, either with a hunting-
and-gathering lifestyle or as farmers or fishermen. Then Western "progress" arrives, along with a lot of Western foods as
well as a less physically challenging lifestyle, and both obesity and diabetes rates soar, with diabetes rates sometimes
approaching 50 percent of the entire population.

As I mentioned earlier, no one has yet figured out exactly
which of the many factors involved is most responsible. Diet
gurus with preconceived notions tend to blame the diabetes

on whichever nutrient their diet has labeled as a villain. Some say it's too much fat. Some say it's too much refined carbohydrate. Some say it's simply too many calories. Some say it's too little exercise. It could also be the increased stress of a modern lifestyle, especially when that lifestyle is strange to those who adopt it.

The answer could be any one of these factors, or a combination of all of them, or it could be something else we haven't discovered yet. But it's a good guess that the change from real foods to highly processed foods that contain both highly refined carbohydrates and a lot of fat is at least partially responsible. One study has shown that among American men, eating a diet high in processed meats such as hot dogs, bacon, salami, or sausage may increase the risk of developing type 2 diabetes. Eating processed meat five or more times per week increased a man's risk of developing type 2 diabetes by nearly 50 percent.

On the other hand, another study showed that eating a lot of salad all year round resulted in a *reduced* rate of diabetes.

Thus until someone proves otherwise, you're apt to be a lot better off if you can eat as many real foods—as opposed to snack foods and preprepared meals—as you can afford. Whole grains have lower glycemic index values than white flour and sugar. Most fresh vegetables contain a lot of fiber, and this both fills you up and contributes to a slower release of sugar into the bloodstream.

Whole foods also contain more vitamins and minerals, which may be stripped away by heavy processing. A real deficiency in some minerals such as chromium and vanadium is known to produce diabetes symptoms. Eating nothing but refined foods could produce a chromium deficiency both because there was no chromium in the refined foods and because digesting carbohydrates requires chromium, which may be lost in the process.

Sure, some manufacturers "fortify" their products with the vitamins and minerals they've removed by refining, and you can also take vitamin pills to make up for the deficiencies in the processed foods. Taking a lot of supplements may help ensure that you have no vitamin and mineral deficiencies, but it's always better to get these nutrients with your food. It's possible that whole foods contain yet-undiscovered substances that might help keep your blood glucose levels on an even keel and thus help forestall the onset of diabetes.

The advantage of getting vitamins from whole foods was shown in a study of beta-carotene—which forms vitamin A in the body—and lung cancer rates. Early studies showed that people who ate a lot of beta-carotene–rich foods had lower rates of lung cancer. So scientists set up a study to investigate the role of beta-carotene supplements on lung cancer rates in smokers, fully expecting that those who were taking the supplements would get less cancer. To their surprise, it turned out that those who took the supplements actually had *higher* rates of lung cancer. Apparently, something that seemed to be protective when eaten as part of a whole food was not protective when given as a supplement.

It's not always easy to eat real foods, especially if you have to eat institutional food or if you're always on the go and the restaurant choices are limited. Traveling on interstates or traveling just as a means of getting from here to there often means you won't find any restaurants except generic fast-food places. Much of what they offer is apt to be high in trans fat and high in fast carbohydrates. Good vegetables in particular are often difficult to find. Thus these places are not ideal for your new way of eating, and you're better off packing your own meals. You can always stop for coffee or tea.

Or bring part of the meal. Cut up raw or blanched vegetbales like carrots, broccoli, cauliflower, pepper, celery, and green beans, and pack them in a cooler. You can either add them to a restaurant dish that offers no fresh vegetables, snack on them between stops, or add a little dressing and some lettuce and olives and make them into a salad.

Sometimes real foods appear to be more expensive, but this is not always true. I recently did an experiment with green beans. I bought some fresh green beans, some frozen green beans, and some canned green beans. I weighed them before and after cooking and compared the results. The cheapest beans turned out to be the frozen, because there was no waste. A pound of frozen beans produced a pound of cooked beans. Next came the fresh beans, which cost the same per pound as the frozen. But there was a little waste, because you pay for stems that you throw away. However, they tasted so much better and offered so many more options—raw, light steaming, or thorough cooking—that the small amount of waste was a minor factor for me. The most expensive by far turned out to be the canned beans, because a large part of the contents consists of water. They also contain a lot of sodium.

So before you conclude that you can't afford fresh foods, do some experimenting to see if that's really true.

Human beings evolved eating real foods, not industrially modifed foods. Thus the chances that our bodies are equipped to deal with real foods are greater than the chances that we can deal with factory foods. Even when there's no proof that a piece of reconstituted meat covered with highly refined white flour and fried in industrially produced vegetable shortening is harmful, your chances would be better with real chicken cooked with olive oil.

Unfortunately, not everyone can escape processed foods all of the time. But escape them as much as you are able and your chances of good health and lower diabetes risks should increase.

find something to do at home that's more interesting than tv

R A T I O N A L E :

Watching TV is associated with higher diabetes rates.

except for lying still or sleeping, there's no activity that burns fewer calories than watching TV.

TV watching is a passive activity. There are exceptions, for instance if you're jumping up and down screaming because your favorite team is winning the Super Bowl, or if you're wrestling with someone over the remote control. But in general, TV watching can put you into a sort of catatonic state. Even sitting in a chair reading requires more calories than watching TV.

Here are a few mostly nonstrenuous activities you might do at home, or nearby, with the number of calories burned by doing them. The actual numbers aren't important, because they differ depending on the size and sex of the person doing the various activities. Large men burn more calories just sitting around than small women do. The figures were calculated based on a 160-pound, 5-foot, 11-inch man, from the Web site *www.caloriesperhour.com.*

What's important is the relative number of calories.

CALORIES BURNED WITH MILD EXERCISE

Sleeping or lying still	67
Watching TV	74
Sitting reading	97
Playing cards or knitting	112
Attending a class	134
Strolling or playing the guitar	149
Washing the dishes	171
Cooking, vacuuming, putting away groceries, playing billiards, or playing the violin	186
Acting or child care while sitting	223
Walking the dog	261
Playing the drums	298
Refinishing furniture or dancing	335
Vigorous child care	372
Square dancing	409

Most people don't think of playing cards or knitting as exercise, but they burn almost one and a half times as many calories as does watching TV. Learn to play the guitar and you're burning twice as many. Take up the drums and you'll burn four times as many calories. Refinish some furniture and you'll not only burn more calories, but you may end up with a profitable business as well.

Vigorous exercise, or simply taking the dog for a walk, is a wonderful thing to do to reduce your risk of diabetes. But trying to avoid totally passive activities like lying on a recliner staring at the ceiling—or watching TV—is important too. Try-

find something to do at home that's more interesting than tv

ing to find something interesting to do when you're at home and the TV is calling your name is just as important as trying to find ways of moving more when you're out and about.

This is especially important if you live in an unsafe urban neighborhood and you're not comfortable coming and going from your home. Can you learn to play a musical instrument? Take up cooking? Babysit for the neighbors? Repaint the living room? Make new curtains? Visit an elderly shut-in?

Almost any activity is better than watching TV.

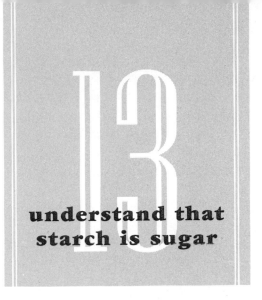

understand that starch is sugar

R A T I O N A L E :

Understanding how starch raises your blood sugar
will help you make wise food choices.

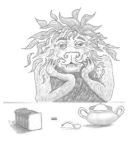

most people associate diabetes with sugar. They think eating too much sugar causes diabetes and that when you have diabetes, you can't eat sugar, but everything else is OK. Unfortunately, some nutritionists and people who manufacture "diabetic foods" and sell "diabetic cookbooks" still think the same thing. They think that sugar is bad and "complex carbohydrates" like starch are good. But it's simply not true.

Sugar is a carbohydrate. As I mentioned before, carbohydrates are the foods that raise your blood sugar. Carbohydrates with a low glycemic index, for example whole foods containing a lot of fiber, raise your blood sugar levels slowly. Carbohydrates with a high glycemic index, for example, glucose and rice cakes, raise your blood sugar much faster.

It may come as a surprise to learn that the glycemic index of sucrose (table sugar) is not especially high. Why is this? It's because sucrose consists of two different sugars, *glucose* and *fructose,* linked together. Scientists call this a *disaccharide,* meaning "two sugars." Glucose is the sugar that your cells use for energy. It has a high glycemic index and, when eaten, raises your blood glucose levels extremely quickly.

Because glucose has such a high glycemic index, it is often the standard by which other foods are compared (the other standard is white bread, which also raises your blood sugar levels quickly, but not quite as quickly as glucose). Glucose is given a glycemic index of 100. Anything with a glycemic index lower than 100 raises your blood sugar more slowly than glucose. Anything with a glycemic index higher than 100 raises your blood sugar even faster than glucose.

Fructose has a low glycemic index and raises your blood glucose levels very slowly. Because sucrose consists of half high–glycemic index glucose (100) and half low–glycemic index fructose (23), its glycemic index is about halfway in between (65).

Then how about starch? Well, starch consists of long chains of glucose linked together like beads on a necklace. Scientists call it a *polysaccharide,* meaning "many sugars." When you eat starchy foods, digestive enzymes in your body break the long chains down into glucose, which has a very high glycemic index.

These enzymes start to work in your mouth. You can even detect the glucose that is released from starch by chewing a starchy food like white bread for a few minutes. You should begin to taste the sweetness.

Scientists used to think that because the glucose chains of

understand that starch is sugar

starch are so long, it would take them a long time to break down, so your blood glucose levels would rise more slowly than they would when you ate a sugar like glucose or sucrose. It turns out, this is not true. Starch breaks down so quickly that it raises your blood glucose levels as fast as table sugar, sometimes even faster because, as I noted, it contains nothing but high–glycemic index glucose.

Foods containing starch—for example, breads—may raise your blood sugar at different rates depending on the other ingredients. For example, French bread, which usually contains only highly milled flour, yeast, salt, and water, has a glycemic index of 95, almost as high as pure glucose. Stone-ground whole-wheat bread—which probably includes some fat as well as coursely ground whole wheat—has a glycemic index of 53. Even very starchy foods like white bread do contain some protein and may be enriched with some vitamins, but they're still primarily starch, which is just long chains of sugar.

This means that if you're trying to keep your consumption of fast carbohydrates down, starchy foods like bread and potatoes and white rice (especially "sticky" rice) and some breakfast cereals are not good choices.

Forget what you've heard about "complex carbohydrates," which is a vague term that has changed in meaning over the past several years. Instead, focus on the glycemic index. In general, whole foods that aren't highly refined have a lot of fiber and low glycemic index values, but this is not always true. Starchy foods like potatoes have relatively little fiber and a lot of starch. When further processed into whipped or mashed potatoes, they raise your blood glucose levels even faster. Highly processed instant mashed potatoes are the worst.

If you become diabetic, you may find that you have to severely curtail your consumption of carbohydrate foods, especially starchy foods with a high glycemic index. That's one good reason to avoid becoming diabetic if you possibly can.

Unfortunately, if you're like a lot of people, starchy foods are the ones you crave. So giving them up completely is hard. If you're trying to reduce your risks of getting diabetes, it's good to cut back on the starchy high-glycemic foods, but this doesn't mean you have to give them up entirely. Just save them for occasional treats.

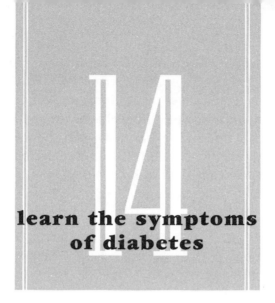

learn the symptoms of diabetes

R A T I O N A L E :

If you're familiar with the symptoms of diabetes,
it's more likely you'll be diagnosed in the early stages,
when the disease may be reversible.

the symptoms of diabetes include excessive thirst, excessive appetite, frequent urination, blurry vision, infections that heal slowly, recurrent yeast infections, unexplained drowsiness or fatigue, unexplained weight gain or loss, and sometimes tingling or pain in the feet or hands (see Table 2).

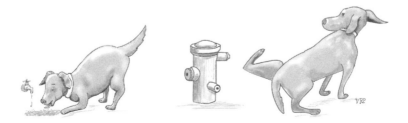

Note that most lists of diabetes symptoms include weight *loss*. This is a symptom of advanced diabetes, such as type 1 diabetes or type 2 diabetes that has progressed quite far. Some people who develop type 2 diabetes report unexplained weight *gain* before they were diagnosed, despite an active lifestyle and careful attention to diet. Another clue that you are at risk is dark pigmentation on the neck or armpits, with the somewhat cumbersome name of *acanthosis nigricans*.

TABLE 2

SYMPTOMS OF TYPE 2 DIABETES

Constant thirst

Frequent urination

Unexplained fatigue

Blurry vision

Unexplained weight loss

Unexplained weight gain, especially around the middle

Tingling or numbness in the hands and/or feet

Constant hunger despite an adequate diet

Unusual drowsiness after meals

Slow healing of wounds

Recurrent yeast infections

Note: Not everyone has all these symptoms. Some people have only one or a few. Some people with type 2 diabetes have no symptoms at all.

Unfortunately, by the time a lot of the symptoms listed in Table 2 appear, the diabetes may be fairly well advanced, and it may not be possible to reverse it simply by losing weight. You may recall that I said that high blood glucose levels for long periods of time can damage your beta cells, the ones that produce insulin. By the time you have real symptoms of diabetes, you may have had high blood glucose levels for years, and some of your beta cells may be irreversibly damaged.

learn the symptoms of diabetes

Some people estimate that about 80 percent of your beta cells have to be damaged before you get these symptoms.

Thus you want to make sure that if you do get type 2 diabetes, you are diagnosed early, before a lot of these symptoms appear.

Factors that increase your risk of type 2 diabetes include the following:

❑ Having prediabetes
❑ Being overweight
❑ Getting little exercise
❑ Being over sixty-five years of age
❑ Having given birth to a baby weighing more than nine pounds
❑ Having a parent or sibling with type 2 diabetes
❑ Having high blood pressure and abnormal blood fat levels
❑ Having dark pigmentation on the neck or armpits (*acanthosis nigricans*)
❑ Belonging to an ethnic group with high diabetes rates (including African American, Hispanic/Latino American, Asian America, Native American, Pacific Islander American, or Arab American).

Note that within these ethnic groups, diabetes rates may differ. For example, Cuban Americans have lower rates than do Mexican Americans; the Dene Indians have relatively low rates and the Pima Indians have high rates.

If your risks are high, see a doctor every year to make sure your blood glucose levels are normal. Official guidelines currently recommend testing for diabetes only every three years, but a blood glucose test is not an expensive test, and if you're at high risk, there's no reason to risk two extra years of high blood glucose levels if you don't have to. If you can't afford a physical exam every year, seek out free diabetes screening tests that are often offered at health fairs or by civic groups.

If you think you see signs that something might be wrong—for example, if you have *acanthosis nigricans* or if you suddenly start putting on weight, especially around your midsection, without any change in your diet or exercise patterns, ask your doctor about doing extra tests for diabetes (see also Tip 24).

If anyone in your family has ever had *hemochromatosis*, an iron-storage disease, and especially if you have a Celtic background (because hemochromatosis is more common in people with this heritage), make sure your doctor checks you for that. If you're a woman and have irregular periods, or trouble with infertility, especially if you also have a weight problem and excess body and facial hair, ask your doctor about *polycystic ovary syndrome, or PCOS.*

When you have your blood glucose level tested, don't accept a simple statement that you don't have diabetes. Ask for the number, and keep track of the numbers through the years. Even if your numbers are still within normal limits, if they're starting to creep up, it's a suggestion that you're at increasing risk for diabetes, and you'll want to increase your efforts to stave it off.

Early detection is one of the most important ways to ensure that you will never get any serious complications from diabetes.

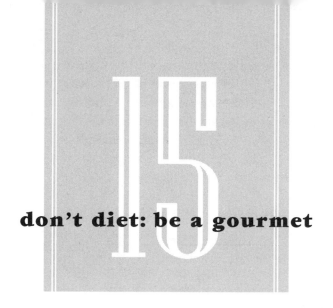

don't diet: be a gourmet

RATIONALE:

If you don't feel deprived, you'll most likely eat less.

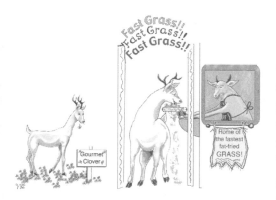

"out of sight, out of mind"? Or "Absence makes the heart grow fonder"? When it comes to diets, I'll cast my vote for the latter. There's nothing like going on a diet to make you become obsessed with food. Every waking moment, you're dreaming of the next meal, thinking of all the tempting treats that are temporarily (you hope) forbidden to you.

The problem with diets is that even if you do eventually

reach your goal weight, you'll crave all those forbidden fruits so much that you'll probably overindulge when you stop the diet and regain all the weight you lost, and then some.

A much better approach is not to think of yourself as being on a diet at all. Instead of viewing yourself as a fat person who is being "punished" by being put on a diet, think of yourself as a thin gourmet (temporarily disguised as a fat person) who is always seeking the best food, the most marvelous tastes, but who, once that food is found, simply tastes a small portion and leaves the rest. The goal of the gourmet is the ultimate taste, not the quantity that can be downed.

Wherever you are, seek out the *best* food, not the largest portions. Order the exotic twelve-dollar appetizer instead of the twelve-dollar all-you-can eat starchy buffet. If you're offered some food, consult your inner thin gourmet. Is this food something I really want? Will it taste really good? Or am I tempted because it's free? Or because it's there? Or because everyone else is having it?

A gourmet doesn't even bother with inferior food like fast-food burgers or fries. Of course, you have to eat a little something regularly, and if fast food is the only thing available at the time, you'll have to make do. But you don't need to order as if you were starving. See what you can do to turn something on the menu into a gourmet's treat—a small one, of course.

Carry special pickles or condiments from a gourmet outlet and add them to a salad. Order some lean meat and spice it up with an interesting Asian sauce you found at a market downtown. Always focus on taste instead of quantity both when eating at home and when eating out.

Learn to savor your food. Eat slowly. Chewing your food thoroughly instead of bolting it down not only improves your digestion but slows the meal down and hence increases the chances that you'll feel full before you've eaten too much. It takes ten or twenty minutes for your stomach to tell your brain that you've eaten enough so the brain can turn off its hunger signals. In addition, chewing seems to help some people feel satisfied after a meal. That's one problem with liquid meals: They provide calories but no chewing.

Think about the taste of what you're eating. Is this the best combination of tastes and mouth sensations that you can imagine? If you've cooked the dish, think of how you could make it even more pleasurable the next time you fix it. If you're eating out, can you guess the exotic ingredients? A gourmet is always trying to improve on the past.

Diets are for other people. Most dieters aren't able to keep the weight off in the long run. But you're different. You're not on a diet. You've embarked on a lifelong quest for small portions of the very best food you can find. You're a gourmet.

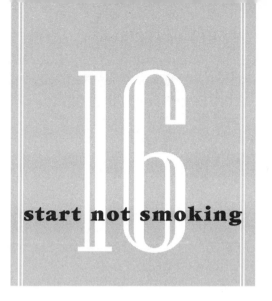

start not smoking

Smoking causes the body to produce the same harmful chemicals that high blood glucose levels do, and smoking increases the incidence of type 2 diabetes.

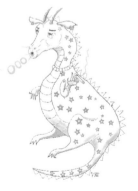

everyone knows that

smoking isn't healthy. It can wreck your lungs. But most people don't know that smoking produces the same harmful protein products that high levels of glucose in the blood do.

When blood glucose levels are elevated for long periods of time, they produce chemical compounds called AGEs, which stands for *advanced glycation end products*. Glucose molecules become attached to proteins in a way that is almost completely irreversible.

This reaction is very similar to the browning of meat, which also produces AGEs. In your body, the proteins that have become AGEs don't work the way they're supposed to. When you get AGEs in your skin, for instance, your skin loses its elasticity, and you're more apt to get wrinkles. When you get AGEs in other organs, they don't work as well, and you can end up with kidney damage or damage to your eyes or other organs.

Some AGEs are formed slowly throughout your life, and one theory of aging is that the AGEs build up and gradually make your whole body less efficient. People with diabetes form AGEs at a faster rate, and thus people with diabetes often age faster than normal.

Cigarette smoking does the same thing. This may be one reason why people who smoke seem to get wrinkled skin at an earlier age than nonsmokers. If you're at risk for diabetes, you're also at risk for accelerated aging and early heart disease. Does it make any sense to increase your risk even more by smoking?

It's also possible that AGEs contribute to the onset of diabetes in people who have diabetes genes. Studies have shown that smoking increases the incidence of type 2 diabetes. One study showed that children whose mothers smoked during pregnancy were up to four times more likely to become diabetic than those whose mothers were nonsmokers.

Obviously, it's not easy to stop smoking once you're already hooked. I can't tell you the best way to stop. But if you possibly can, stop smoking and slow down your AGEs and your aging, as well as reducing your risk of getting type 2 diabetes.

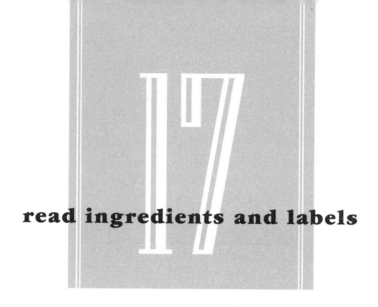

read ingredients and labels

R A T I O N A L E :

It's important to know what's in the food you're eating and to reject any foods that contain substances you're trying to avoid.

apples and squashes don't come with nutritional labels. And in general, fresh apples and squashes are better choices than TV dinners. But most of us buy some foods and ingredients in a packaged form. When you do, it's important to know exactly what you're getting. Thus it's important to learn how to read ingredient lists and labels.

When reading the list of ingredients for a product, the most important thing to know is that manufacturers are required to list the ingredients by weight. Thus an ingredient list that starts with sugar means that there's more sugar in the product than anything else. A product in which sugar is the last ingredient might contain only a dash of sugar.

Manufacturers sometimes list the ingredients in a misleading way. For example, a sugary product might list *whole wheat flour, sugar* (meaning *sucrose), high-fructose corn syrup, molasses,* and *maple syrup* as the first ingredients. Everything but the flour is a kind of sugar, but by listing them separately, no one sugar makes up the bulk of the product, so it may appear that there's more flour than sugars, when in fact the combined sugars make up the bulk of the product. Also, manufacturers sometimes use less common forms of sugar such as *rice syrup, treacle,* or *sorghum,* and you might not realize what they are. The producers are not necessarily trying to confuse you; there might be an economic reason to use unusual sugars. But you need to understand that if you're trying to limit some particular type of food, you need to learn to identify it in various different forms.

If you see an ingredient you're not familiar with, either reject the product or write down the name and look it up. You can keep a list of these unfamiliar ingredients along with your shopping list so you can understand them when you see them in other products. Just because a name isn't familiar doesn't necessarily mean that it's harmful. But it's better if you know what you're eating.

Sometimes the lists of ingredients are hidden under flaps. This tends to be common with some bars such as "energy bars" or "nutrition bars." These products often have names that suggest that they're healthy foods. But if you read the ingredient list, you may find that they contain primarily a lot of sugar, some cheap form of fat, some refined protein, and a few vitamins that you could get just as easily, and a lot more cheaply, in a daily multivitamin pill. Such bars might come in handy in a situation in which you are simply unable to stop for a meal—for example, if you're fleeing from bandits while crossing the Gobi Desert. Otherwise, they're basically very expensive candy bars.

The other useful label on packaged foods is the food label. Figure 6 shows a typical food label. Most of the label is clear.

For one serving size, it shows the total calories and the amount of fat, sodium, carbohydrate, and protein.

Nutrition Facts

Serving Size 3 pieces (15g)
Servings Per Container 15

Amount Per Serving

Calories 60   Calories from Fat 25

	% Daily Value*
Total Fat 3g	5%
Saturated Fat 0.5g	3%
Polyunsaturated Fat 0.5g	
Monounsaturated Fat 1.0g	
Cholesterol 0mg	0%
Sodium 110mg	5%
Total Carbohydrate 9g	3%
Dietary Fiber 1g	4%
Sugars 0.5g	
Protein 2g	

Vitamin A 0%	•	Vitamin C 0%
Calcium 0%	•	Iron 4%

* Percent Daily Values are based on a 2,000 calorie diet. Your daily values may be higher or lower depending on your calorie needs:

	Calories:	2,000	2,500
Total Fat	Less than	65g	60g
Sat. Fat	Less than	20g	25g
Cholesterol	Less than	300mg	300mg
Sodium	Less than	2,400mg	2,400mg
Total Carbohydrate		300g	375g
Dietary Fiber		25g	30g

INGREDIENTS: UNBLEACHED ENRICHED WHEAT FLOUR [FLOUR, MALTED BARLEY, NIACIN, REDUCED IRON, THIAMIN, MONONITRATE (VITAMIN B1), RIBOFLAVIN (VITAMIN B2), FOLIC ACID], PARTIALLY HYDROGENATED SOYBEAN OIL, OAT FIBER, DEXTROSE, SALT, YEAST.

Figure 6. A nutrition label. Note that the serving size for this hypothetical product is three pieces. If you ate fifteen pieces, you'd be getting five times as much of the amounts stated on the label per serving: for example, 300 hundred calories and 125 grams of fat. Note also that the label gives the Daily Values for a diet containing either 2000 or 2500 calories, but the % Daily Values are based only on the 2000-calorie diet. If you eat more or less, your percentages may be more or less, as well.

This hypothetical product also appears to contain 1 gram of trans fat. There are two signs that the product contains trans fat. First, the ingredients include partially hydrogenated soybean oil. Second, the saturated, polyunsaturated, and monounsaturated fats total 2 grams, but the total fat is 3 grams. Hence there's about 1 gram of trans fat (I say *about* because some of these numbers may be rounded).

You can also estimate the amount of starch in this product. It contains 1 gram of fiber and 0.5 gram of sugar. But there are 9 grams of total carbohydrate. Hence the product contains 7.5 grams (9–1.5) of nonsugar, nonfiber carbohydrate, that is, some kind of starch. Some labels even tell you how much soluble fiber and how much insoluble fiber.

The total fat and carbohydrate may be broken down into different types of fat and carbohydrate. Thus the fat may list saturated fat, monounsaturated fat, and polyunsaturated fat (see Tip 6). In the near future, labels should also list the amount of trans fat. For now, you can estimate the trans fat content by adding up the total grams of saturated, monounsaturated, and polyunsaturated fats and subtracting that from the total fat. If there's anything left over, that's trans fat. For example, let's say the label says there are 5 grams of total fat. If the label lists 1 gram of saturated fat, 1.5 grams of monounsaturated fat, and 1.5 grams of polyunsaturated fat, that totals 4 grams. But there are 5 grams of total fat. So there must be 1 gram of trans fat.

The carbohydrate may also be broken down into fiber (see Tip 4) and sugars. Anything that is left over is probably starch. For example, let's say the label lists 12 grams of carbohydrate. It also lists 2 grams of fiber and 6 grams of sugars (these could be any of various sugars). That makes 8 grams, but there are 12 grams total, so the product must include 4 grams of non-sugar, nonfiber carbohydrate, which usually means some kind of starch.

One important thing to understand about a food label is the portion size. The various amounts of nutrients refer to the amounts *found in the portion size listed on the label.* Sometimes the portion sizes are quite small, so you might think you aren't getting many calories or grams of fat or carbohydrate when you eat the product. But if the portion size is a quarter of a cup and you usually eat a cup of the product, you'll be getting four times as much of everything as stated on the label.

Sometimes manufacturers use tiny portion sizes to make their products appear to be low fat or low carb or whatever it is they're touting. Also keep this in mind when you're comparing products. Product A contains five grams of fat in two tablespoons, and product B contains ten grams of fat in four tablespoons. Just glancing at the label, you might think product A had less fat, but they both contain the same amount.

Another important thing to note is that the percentages of the *daily value* (the amount estimated to be important for you to eat each day) are based on a person eating a 2000-calorie diet. If you eat more or less than 2000 calories, your requirements will be proportionately more or less. If you're eating 2500 calories, you need to multiply the percentages by 2500/2000, or 1.25. If you're eating only 1500 calories a day, you need to multiply them by 1500/2000, or 0.75.

Note that if the numbers don't always add up exactly, it may be because the manufacturers have rounded their numbers off: 1.46 could be rounded up to 1.5 or rounded down to 1.

These are the essential things you need to know about a food label. In my book *The First Year—Type 2 Diabetes,* I discuss some more subtle points about the food label that people who need to count their carbohydrates very carefully need to know. When you don't have diabetes, you don't usually need to be quite as accurate in your nutritional counts.

Using the food label should help you to choose packaged foods that satisfy your needs. If you're interested in increasing the fiber in your diet, pay attention to the fiber content of these foods. If you want to avoid trans fats, try to calculate the trans fat content.

Of course, the fewer boxed and processed foods you eat, the better. And whole foods often don't have food labels, although some health food stores and co-ops have nutritional labels on their bulk bins. It's usually enough to know general properties of foods—for example, that fruits usually contain a lot of soluble fiber and almost no fat, and whole grains usually contain a lot of insoluble fiber. If you want to know the particulars, they are easily found in books listing the nutritional content of foods or on the U.S. Department of Agriculture's Internet nutrient resource (currently at *http://www.nal.usda.gov/fnic/cgi-bin/nut_search.plf*). If the

URL has changed, you can type *nutritional content of food,* or similar terms, into a Web search engine to find it or other useful sites.

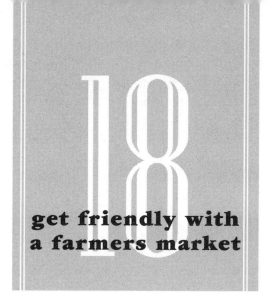

get friendly with a farmers market

The best way to ensure that you'll eat a lot of fiber-rich vegetables and fruits is to make sure they taste delicious. Freshly picked food always tastes the best, and the freshest food is often found at farmers markets.

remember, you're a gourmet. You want only the freshest, tastiest foods. Huge portions of canned peas or macaroni and processed cheese are for other people. You're looking for something better. You've already tasted canned peas and macaroni and cheese, and you know what they taste like. You're looking for something new.

When you go to the supermarket, you'll usually find only one or two varieties of any particular fruit or vegetable, often only one. Apples tend to be Macintosh or Delicious. Sometimes there are a few more varieties of apples, but not many. Strawberries are usually called *strawberries*, with no indication of their origin or type.

But in fact there are many many different varieties of most

fruits and vegetables. Many of them are too fragile for shipping long distances, or for storage for long periods of time. Hence you can usually find them only if you buy directly from the producer. I once went to a local apple orchard that offered thirty or so different varieties of apples, including some of my favorites like Northern Spy and Pound Sweet, and some that I'd never heard of, like Blue Pearmain. I bought one of each.

When you buy direct from the producer, you can inquire about the variety of strawberry or lettuce or broccoli that you're buying. If you find you like one variety better than another, you can make sure to ask about it in the future.

Produce bought from a farmers market is also fresher, sometimes even picked on the morning it is sold. The same usually applies to a roadside farm stand. The advantage of a farmers market is that you get a larger variety of produce from a large variety of farms. Sometimes such markets also sell locally raised, hormone-free meat, unusual cheeses, fresh fish, and various baked goods as well.

If you live in an area with a nearby farmers market, you're in luck. But not everyone does. If not, make inquiries (a federal Extension office or the local chamber of commerce would be a good place to start) and see if there's one within driving distance. Then turn a shopping day into a weekend outing. Many such markets include live music, animal exhibits, and other events that children would enjoy. Make sure you work some activity into your outing. Just walking around the market should provide some exercise. Maybe you can walk even farther and explore the neighborhood, especially if it's in a rural or suburban area.

What if you're in an inner-city area, there are no farmers markets nearby, and you don't have a car? You're surely not the only person who might benefit from a combination of fresh vegetables and fruits and a nice outing to the country. Talk with a local social service agency to see if they could start a program to rent a van or bus and take a group of you to a

get friendly with a farmers market

farmers market once a month, or once a week if you're lucky. You could also stop at a discount supermarket on the way back to stock up on staples that might be more expensive at your local convenience store.

Instead of going to a farmers market, another option would be to have some of the farmers market come to you. If you could get enough neighbors who wanted to buy fresh produce but weren't able to get to a market, you could see if someone was willing to bring a truckload of fresh produce to your neighborhood—either the farmers themselves or a few people who could take orders and bring the produce to a central location for distribution.

Another option is a relatively new concept called Community Supported Agriculture, or CSA. This requires you to pay in advance and hence would be difficult if you're living from paycheck to paycheck. But if you can come up with the cash, it's a good deal. You pay a lump sum in the spring. A farmer uses your money for seeds and fertilizers, and then throughout the spring and summer you get fresh produce from the farm.

Both farmers markets and CSA may have programs to help those with low incomes buy fresh produce at a discount. Some take food stamps or special coupons designed for this purpose. The WIC Farmers' Market Nutrition Program is active in about forty states and Indian Tribal Organizations, in addition to Washington, DC, and Guam. Ask if such a program is available in your state.

By shopping at a farmers market, you're also helping farmers by avoiding the costs of the middleman. So you're not only doing yourself a favor, but you're helping someone else. And remember, you're a gourmet, and you want the best food, the tastiest, the freshest, and the greatest variety. The best way to get this kind of food is from the people who grow it—at a farmers market.

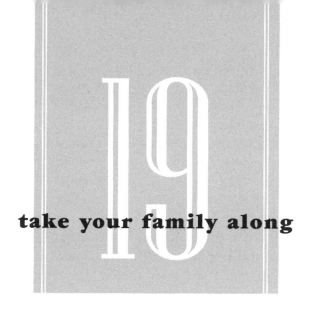

take your family along

R A T I O N A L E :

It's difficult to stick to a healthy way of eating if you're
the only one who's eating that way. A diet that lowers
your risk of diabetes is a healthy diet for everyone, and
the rest of your family should benefit as well.

if you think you're at risk for diabetes, it means
you think you have diabetes genes. That means your children
are also at risk of having the same genes. There is no gift you
could give them that is more valuable than the gift of growing up with a healthy diet so they think that eating a diet filled
with vegetables and other real foods is the normal way to eat.

The same is true of exercise. It is a precious gift to show
your children through example that getting exercise can be
fun—by including them as much as possible in the active per-
suits you have chosen—instead of giving them the idea that
growing up means the freedom to spend more hours on the
couch watching TV.

Taking your family along on your new eating adventure

will also make it easier for you. If you've decided that potato chips have too many trans fats and too many fast carbohydrates for you, it's a lot easier to avoid eating them if there aren't any in the house.

As with starting the many small steps that will reduce your risks of type 2 diabetes, starting a new lifestyle for your family is probably best done in small steps. If you come home one day after work and tell the family that you've sold the TV, you're not going to buy any more sodas or potato chips, and everyone has to get up at dawn to play touch football, you'll probably just start a mutiny, and the kids may go out and rent new parents.

So go slowly. You might want to start by example. Make little changes in your own lifestyle. Prepare especially tasty new foods using your new guidelines, and see if anyone else wants a taste. If they like what they taste, make it for everyone next time. If not, see how you can modify it to appeal to their tastebuds while keeping to your new cooking guidelines.

The first time you start a new activity designed to help you move more, try to make it an especially interesting one. No kid is apt to want to join you on a treadmill or a stair-stepping machine. But what if you decide to learn how to skate? Ride a horse? Learn to tap dance? Learn to rock climb? Or just explore a new hiking trail?

Even so, some family members may be resistant at first. But what if they notice you've begun to lose some weight and your muscles are beginning to firm up? If they're not satisfied with their own builds, they may start to ask how you managed to change.

You may simply want to set the rules. No more potato chips in this house. No sodas with dinner. If you want to rent a video, you have to walk to the store to get it. They'll probably whine a lot, but they'll get used to it. And if they find that Dad's or Mom's new "unfair" regime is making them slimmer and stronger than they used to be, they'll be glad even if they hate to admit it.

Even if they don't pay attention now, setting a good example for your children may be a gift for the future when they could begin to have weight problems themselves. If you're young yourself and don't yet have kids, think of making your parents proud by eating better food and being more active. Your parents might even begin to imitate *you*.

Maybe even your friends will begin to notice the changes in you and ask what you're doing to make yourself slimmer and stronger. If you live in a neighborhood that includes other people who are also apt to be at risk of diabetes, you could organize a group to discuss the kinds of changes that have worked for you and help other people reduce their risks of diabetes too.

It's hard to change all by yourself. The larger the group of people who are trying to make a change, the easier it should be.

keep an eye on your fats and blood pressure

RATIONALE:

Having high levels of triglycerides in your blood along with low levels of HDL, high blood pressure, and an apple shape suggests that you may have insulin resistance, which usually results in type 2 diabetes. Knowing your risks should help you take action early.

as I outlined in the introduction (see Figure 1), type 2 diabetes usually starts with insulin resistance. You recall that insulin resistance means that even though you may be producing plenty of insulin, for some yet-unknown reason, it doesn't work very well. No one understands yet exactly how insulin resistance works, but it is known to cause a lot of metabolic diseases, including type 2 diabetes, polycystic ovary syndrome, and something called by various names, most commonly *metabolic syndrome X,* or often just syndrome X.

Syndrome X includes insulin resistance and the resulting high insulin levels, an "apple shape" (most of your weight in your stomach), high levels of triglycerides (fats), high blood pressure, and low levels of high-density lipoprotein (HDL), the so-called good cholesterol that reduces your risks of heart disease by ferrying cholesterol from the circulation to the liver for disposal.

People who have syndrome X have a very high risk of heart disease. And because the syndrome includes insulin resistance, if they *also* have a genetic defect in the beta cells that keeps them from producing a whole lot of insulin (review Figure 2), they often progress to prediabetes (review Figure 5) and then to full-blown diabetes.

It's difficult to measure insulin resistance directly. It can be done, but the test is very time-consuming and expensive and is usually done only in research laboratories. Hence your doctor can't simply order an insulin resistance test for you whenever you have a physical exam. However, if you have several of the factors that go along with insulin resistance, for example, an apple shape as well as high blood pressure, high levels of triglycerides, and low levels of HDL—all things that can be measured fairly easily when you have lab work done—this is strongly suggestive that you might have insulin resistance as well.

If you do, you're at high risk for heart disease as well as diabetes, and you should work hard to bring all your lab results—as well as your apple shape—back into healthy ranges. If you work at this *before* you've actually developed any signs of diabetes, you'll still have 100 percent of your beta cells, and your chances of keeping your blood sugar normal will be much, much better.

In fact, not everyone with the signs of syndrome X will progress to type 2 diabetes even if they do nothing to change their way of life. But many will have heart attacks even though their blood glucose levels are normal. Thus working to change your way of life to reduce your syndrome X symptoms will be good for your health, even if it turns out you don't have the diabetes genes after all.

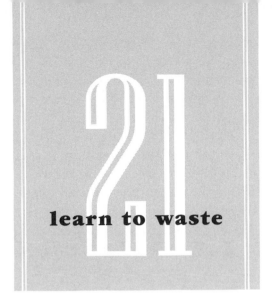

learn to waste

RATIONALE:

Not wasting food may seem like the moral high road, but it can also lead to obesity.

many of you were probably raised as members in full standing of the Clean Plates Club. "Think of the starving children in China" (or India or Armenia or Africa, depending on where the famine of the time was occurring), you were admonished, as you puzzled to know how in the world finishing all of Aunt Maud's turnip casserole could possibly help those poor little starving children halfway across the globe.

Unfortunately, even if you were never really strong supporters of the Clean Plates Club, those childhood sermons probably took root somewhere in your brain, and wasting food continues to seem like a sin. But in fact, when you were a kid, you were right. Eating everything on your plate will have absolutely no effect whatsoever on the nutritional level of people somewhere else in the world. But it will have a large effect on your waistline.

Thus one of the first steps you have to take when you start your new way of eating is to learn to waste. Send back your membership card in the Clean Plates Club. Tell them to stop sending you literature. If you're served at a restaurant or by someone else at a party, eat what you want, and leave the rest. If the High Muckety-Muck of the National Clean Plates Club happens to pass your table and give a gasp of amazement, stick your tongue out at her. You're no longer a member.

Another problem is the family member or friend who keeps urging you to eat more. "Oh come on, you can eat that last bit of stuffing. It's too small to wrap up for tomorrow." If they want to get rid of it, they can eat it themselves—or give it to the dog, or start raising pigs. You've got better things to do than to serve as a garbage disposal for all your family and friends. If that's always been your role, it will take a while for others to get accustomed to the New You. But that's their problem. Don't let them subvert your new way of eating.

I spent too many years as a starving graduate student; when I saw free food, I thought I should eat as much as possible, because I didn't know how much I'd have the next day. This habit is hard to break. In cases like this, you have to remind yourself that by eating more than you need at any one time, you may be saving money in the short run, but you'll lose money in the long run, because medical care is more expensive than food.

I sometimes think one reason rich people tend to be thinner than poor people is because rich people know that good food will always be available to them. There's no need to stock up now. Pretend you're a rich person, even if you're not. Remember you're a gourmet as well. Taste a little of this and a little of that, but only the best that is offered. Ignore the rest.

If you still have trouble not eating as much as you can when the food is "free," try to avoid all-you-can-eat buffets. As a lifelong member of the Tight Wallets Club, I've always had trouble not eating the maximal amount I can stuff into my stomach if I'm paying a fixed price at such buffets. I'm slowly learning, but it's hard. This urge to "stock up" when food is plentiful is not limited to people at all-you-can-eat buffets. Some non-industrialized hunting-and-gathering people eat themselves into a stupor when they're offered all they can eat. Apparently the drive to fill up when the food is available is universal.

Throwing away food when you've always been frugal is extremely difficult. I've never understood those diet books that tell you to start off by going through your pantry and tossing all the food that doesn't conform to their diet plan. What? Throw away perfectly good food?

One way to help get over your anxiety at throwing away food is to start a compost pile. Obviously, composting is a tad difficult if you live in a high-rise apartment. But if you live in the suburbs or in a rural area, you should be able to find a suitable spot for a compost pile. When you have a compost pile, you can throw away leftover plant foods without great pangs of guilt. They're going to turn into something useful, so you haven't wasted them at all.

Not only that, but turning the piles periodically provides a lot of free exercise. They're also a great way to dispose of grass clippings, and raking up the clippings and carrying them to the compost pile will also give you a little more use of your muscles.

If you have a garden, the compost will increase the yield of the garden. If not, you can give the good brown compost to a neighbor who gardens. Maybe you'll even get some nice, fresh homegrown vegetables in return. If no one in your area gardens, you can spread the compost on your lawn instead of using chemical fertilizer. The grass will grow a lot faster and then you'll have to mow it more often. And that's more good exercise for you.

With or without a compost pile, wasting food may be difficult for you. But keep the long-term consequences in mind. Wasting a little food now may save your life for many years. Which is more important?

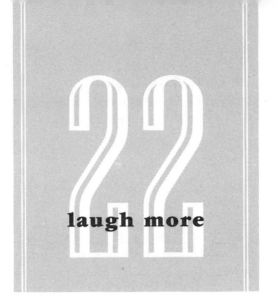

laugh more

R A T I O N A L E :

Laughing reduces stress. Stress increases insulin resistance and thus could contribute to the onset of type 2 diabetes.

when you're under any kind of stress—and this can be physical stress like fighting a kangaroo or mental stress like knowing your taxes are due tomorrow and you haven't even balanced your checkbook for three months—your body produces what are called *stress hormones.*

These stress hormones trigger something called the *fight-or-flight response.* The hormones cause a lot of different reactions that prepare your body to either fight a danger—such as a very small wimpy guy who has threatened you—or to run away from a danger—such as a very large muscular guy who has threatened you.

Your heart rate increases, thus pumping more blood to your brain so you can think quickly, and you stop digesting food, which isn't your first need when you're fighting or fleeing. Also, your body puts more glucose and fatty acids into the blood so you'll have a lot of extra energy to use during the crisis.

The stress hormones that cause all these effects are also called *counterregulatory hormones.* They oppose the action of insulin, meaning they increase insulin resistance. In the short run, this is good, because it causes all the effects I've mentioned, and more. But if your stress levels remain high for a long time, you may be increasing your insulin resistance for no good reason.

Some factors that have been shown recently to increase diabetes rates include:

❑ Caffeine
❑ Gum disease
❑ Chronic lack of sleep
❑ Snoring

Caffeine is known to increase the level of adrenaline, one of the stress hormones. Infections usually increase insulin resistance. And one study showed that people who chronically got between four and six and a half hours of sleep a night had increased insulin resistance. No one understands why snoring increases diabetes rates; obesity—which is often associated with snoring—was not the explanation.

If you've already got a little insulin resistance because of having diabetes genes, and you've got a little more because you're overweight, having the extra insulin resistance from stress hormones may be just enough to send you into a diabetic range.

Laughing is a good way to reduce stress. So anything you can do to increase the amount of time you spend laughing and decrease the time you spend worrying will be beneficial for your general health as well as reducing your risks of diabetes.

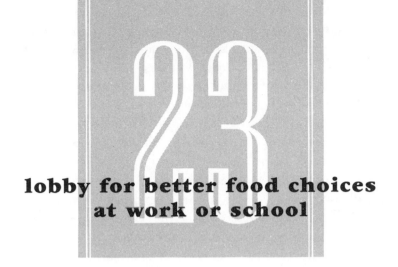

lobby for better food choices at work or school

RATIONALE:

It's easier to follow a sensible diet if you have sensible choices at work or school as well as at home.

when you're at home, you're pretty much in control of what you eat. You can buy the foods you should be eating and leave the junk at the store. But if you work in an office or factory, or if you're at school, it can be much more difficult to follow your new way of eating.

One problem is temptation. Some workplaces provide free snacks for their employees, and many of these snacks are sweet and tempting but full of calories, highly refined carbohydrates, and trans fats.

The other problem is simply availability at mealtimes. Your school or employer may have a cafeteria that serves mostly the kind of food many people want—namely, fast food or breaded and fried foods with chips and maybe a little iceberg lettuce (the least nutritious variety of lettuce). Or maybe the office always sends out for lunch, and the places the other employees choose each day may have limited choices: sandwiches of some kind with chips or fries; or pizza; or takeout Asian foods.

Of course you can always bring your own food. But that means extra work every morning when you're in a rush, and it doesn't solve the problem of temptation.

If you're in such a workplace situation, you're probably not the only person who could benefit from healthier snacks and lunches. If so, get together with some other employees and lobby your employer for some healthier choices.

By *healthier choices* I don't mean just carrot and celery sticks for snacks and a humdrum salad bar for lunch. Given a choice of carrot and celery sticks or a delicious chocolate doughnut, I'm afraid that before my diabetes diagnosis, I would have opted for the doughnut every time. What I mean is *delicious* alternatives. You and the others might have to use your imagination here to make suggestions to the employer or the employer's food service. For example, instead of plain old celery, they could offer celery sticks with unusual cheeses, a different cheese each day; or slices of pears sprinkled with allspice; or fresh apple slices topped with a little hazelnut butter. You could have a contest to see who could bring in the most interesting vegetable snack.

If your employer has a cafeteria, talk with the people who plan the meals to see if they can offer not just salads or an interesting salad bar but cooked foods that don't use a lot of processed ingredients or trans fats. Ask if they could provide broiled meats and lightly steamed vegetables, without sauces. Ask if they'd be willing to offer smaller servings for lower prices. Ask if they could offer brown rice as well as white, or lentils and other legumes instead of potatoes (and foods made from them) all the time.

It might be more difficult to come up with good solutions if everyone sends out for lunch at the same place. You don't want to insist that everyone eat your kind of food if they're determined to eat themselves into an early grave by having nothing but cheeseburgers and supersized fries and colas every day. Maybe you could seek out fascinating alternative places and pick up some food from those places on your way to work. They might get interested in what you're eating and agree to try it a couple of days a week. Anything is better than nothing.

It may take a lot of work, and probably a certain amount of time, before you are always offered healthy options at work, but it's worth the effort. You'll be helping other people become healthier as well as helping yourself

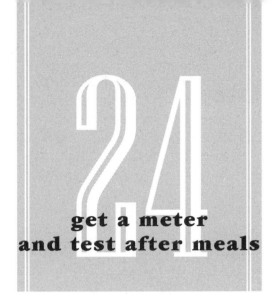

**get a meter
and test after meals**

R A T I O N A L E :

It's easiest to treat type 2 diabetes in the early stages
when your blood glucose levels go up only after meals.
If your medical system won't test this regularly,
you can do it yourself.

go back and look at Figure 5 again. You may remember that I described how type 2 diabetes usually progresses. In the very early stages, your blood glucose levels may be quite normal when you're fasting, or before meals. But when you eat, they go too high.

Your doctor may test your blood sugar levels to make sure you don't have diabetes, but doctors usually test only your *fasting* levels, meaning your blood glucose levels in the morning before you've had anything to eat. This means they could tell you that every thing was hunky-dory, no problem, when in fact your blood sugar was going high after every meal.

In some people, this situation goes on for years. Because high blood glucose levels can damage your beta cells, by

ignoring the condition in its earliest stages, you may be causing unnecessary harm. In addition, high blood glucose levels
can cause AGEs (see Tip 16). By ignoring the early stages of
diabetes, you may be letting your body produce a lot of AGEs,
which can cause faster aging as well as complications such as
damage to your nerves and eyes.

Your doctor can also test you after meals. Usually when
they do this, it's a more formal test called the *glucose tolerance
test,* or GTT. In this test, the doctor measures your blood glucose level and then gives you a sweet drink. Then your blood
glucose level is measured at intervals for a certain period of
time. If two hours later your blood glucose levels are over 200
mg/dL, you are considered to have diabetes. If they're under
140 at two hours, you're considered to be normal. Intermediate levels may indicate prediabetes.

However, the health care system is very much concerned
with keeping costs down, always talking about the cost/ben-
efit ratio of screening people for diabetes when they don't
have symptoms, and many insurance companies won't let
doctors prescribe a GTT unless there is a compelling reason
to do so. Current recommendations include testing fasting levels every three years for people who might be at risk. This
means you could go for more than two years with high fasting blood glucose levels and not know it, and even more
years with normal fasting levels and high levels after meals,
thus increasing your chances of developing complications.

If you think you are at risk for type 2 diabetes and your
health care system won't test you regularly, you can buy a
blood glucose meter and test yourself. The meters cost about
a hundred dollars, and they use disposable test strips that cost
about seventy-five cents each. But if you look around, you
can often find a special offer of a free meter when you buy a
certain number of test strips. Don't buy more than you need,
though, because they have expiration dates.

When I suggested testing yourself after meals, I certainly

get a meter and test after meals

don't mean after every meal. Not even every day. Or every week. Just occasionally, to make sure. If your family has a history of diabetes, it might make sense to test everyone occasionally, maybe once or twice a year. Those with a weight problem might want to test a little more often.

Testing yourself with a meter does mean pricking your finger with a special spring-loaded device, and yes it does hurt just a tiny bit. But it's a small price to pay for the enormous benefit you can gain from learning you're headed in the direction of diabetes before it's too late.

Here's an additional benefit of testing yourself after meals. If you find that your blood glucose levels are *normal* both before and after meals, you'll know you're *not* in the early stages of diabetes. This should reduce your stress levels, which should reduce your levels of stress hormones, which should reduce your chances of developing diabetes in the future, a sort of virtuous circle.

I won't give detailed instructions for how to use a meter. I go into more detail in my book *The First Year—Type 2 Diabetes*. See if you can find it at your library and read the part about buying and using a meter. Or just follow the instructions in the booklet that comes along with your meter.

If you're only going to use the test strips occasionally, you might want to get together with a friend and share a meter and a box of test strips (they *are* expensive, and your insurance isn't apt to pay for a meter and test strips for someone who hasn't already been diagnosed with diabetes). Just one caveat: *Never never* share a needle with someone else because of the dangers of spreading AIDS or hepatitis or other diseases that are spread by exchanging blood. You're unlikely to be at risk if you share a finger pricker and change needles every time. But just to be extra careful, think of it as being like a toothbrush. If you're going to share a meter, make sure to get your own finger pricker, label it carefully, and make sure you use your own every time.

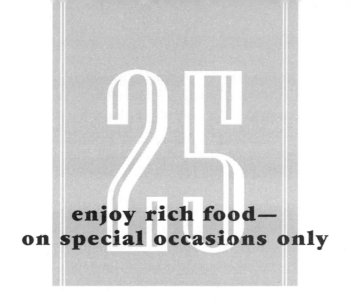

enjoy rich food—
on special occasions only

RATIONALE:

It's better to treat yourself *occasionally* with the rich foods you enjoy than to deprive yourself totally and then give up on your new way of eating.

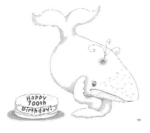

most cultures have special festive foods that they serve on feast days. These foods often have religious or cultural significance as well as being especially tasty. They are often heavy on sweeteners and fat, ingredients that are sometimes scarce in everyday foods.

In some non-Westernized cultures, people may eat tremendous amounts of these festive foods on holidays. But they don't get fat. The important concept here is *on holidays.* On regular days, they eat very plain food: rice with a few vegetables and an occasional piece of meat or egg; rice and beans; fish and seal meat; starchy underground vegetables; simple stews.

What is different about our culture is that festive holiday foods are available for us year-round, every day. They're no longer a treat. We slurp down ice cream and chocolate sauce while we're watching TV, hardly noticing what we're eating. Cheesecake is as common as bread and butter used to be. Croissants, apparently not rich enough as they were served in France, are stuffed with a variety of fattening extras and eaten on daily coffee breaks.

Think of what used to be involved to make strawberry ice cream, which in some homes was served only on the Fourth of July. First, you had to raise the cow. Assuming you already had the cow, you had to milk her the day before and let the cream rise to the top of the pail. Then you skimmed off the cream.

Next you went to the icehouse for some ice that you'd packed in sawdust the winter before. I've never cut ice from a pond myself, but I understand it's a backbreaking job. You had to saw blocks of ice from the pond, then lift them onto a sleigh, drive the sleigh to the icehouse, lift the blocks out into the icehouse, and pack them with sawdust.

After you'd chipped the ice into small pieces with an ice pick, you went to pick some strawberries. Oh yes, I forgot. First you had to grow the strawberries, which meant a lot of work to keep them free from weeds and bugs.

Now you had your cream, your ice, and your strawberries. You probably bought sugar from the store. If not, you'd have to make your own maple sugar, another labor-intensive chore. You probably bought your salt.

Mom boiled up a custard (oh yes, first she had to gather eggs from the henhouse), added the strawberries, and poured it into the ice cream maker. Now everyone in the family took a turn at turning the paddle. As the ice cream got thicker and thicker, the paddle got more and more difficult to turn. Father probably took the last turns, when the ice cream was thickest and the paddle was really difficult to move.

enjoy rich food—on special occasions only

Finally the ice cream was done. If you were lucky, you got an advance taste by licking the paddles. The taste must have been incredible. Fresh milk, fresh berries, and a dish you hadn't had for a year. Needless to say, when the ice cream was finally served at the end of the meal, everyone savored every bite.

And now what do you do? Drive to a convenience store, buy a quart of ice cream, and take it home without a thought. It doesn't taste half as good as ice cream in your great-great-grandmother's day probably tasted. And because it doesn't taste as good, you probably eat even more, trying to substitute for the lack of quality by mechanically eating spoonful after spoonful while you're doing something else.

You want to replicate, as much as possible, the experiences your great-great-grandparents had when they got special holiday treats. Avoid rich foods most of the time. Then, on special holidays and other reasons for celebration, pull out all the stops. Don't settle for a piece of dry cake or some run-of-the mill packaged cookies. Get the best (always remember that you're a gourmet). Eat reasonable amounts. And savor every bite.

Then go back to your simpler everyday way of eating. You know you're not giving up the rich stuff forever. You can remember the last holiday and look forward to the next. Sometimes the anticipation is even better than the actual meal itself.

They say that hunger is the best sauce. The same is true of hunger for special foods. By avoiding them most of the time, you'll increase your pleasure when you do eat them. And gourmets are always looking for ways to increase their pleasure in eating. Gourmets enjoy their food.

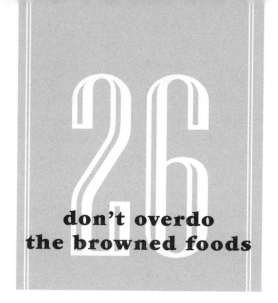

don't overdo the browned foods

R A T I O N A L E :

Browned foods may contain AGEs that could increase your risk of diabetes.

you may recall how AGEs (advanced glycation end products) from cigarette smoking (see Tip 16) or from high blood glucose levels in people with diabetes may cause accelerated aging. Some research has suggested that AGEs from the food you eat may have the same effect.

AGEs are caused when sugars and proteins react together under dry conditions at high temperatures. Scientists call this the *Maillard reaction*. Chefs call it *browning*. Cooks often treat food in ways that encourage browning, such as frying or roasting at high temperatures to encourage browning of the outer layers of meat. Broiling also results in browning, and broiled poultry skin is especially high in AGEs (more than a hundred-fold higher than uncooked). Adding a sugary sauce, for example, barbecue sauce, to meat before cooking causes even more browning. Even bread crusts include some AGEs, as does roasted coffee. On the other hand, moisture discourages the formation of AGEs, so boiled foods don't contain very many. But microwaving food produces AGEs even when the foods don't turn brown. Warming milk in the microwave, for example, increases the AGE level by two or three times.

Browning reactions tend to improve the flavor of food, and not only good cooks but Western food manufacturers have taken advantage of this fact to increase the appeal of food by encouraging browning, for example, by adding sugar to crusts and sauces so they'll brown more.

Studies have shown that when you feed human volunteers foods that are high in AGEs, the levels of AGEs in their blood increase dramatically. In people with normal kidney function, many of the AGEs are excreted in the urine, but some remain.

When researchers fed diabetes-prone mice a low-AGE diet, 60 percent of the mice were diabetes-free after fourteen months. But when they fed another group of mice regular feed that included ten times more AGEs, more than 90 percent of the mice developed diabetes within three months.

Another study showed that a low-AGE diet resulted in a decrease in insulin resistance. If you already have some insulin resistance because of diabetes genes, any decrease would be a good thing.

I know of no studies relating the AGE content of food to the incidence of diabetes in humans. But it's certainly something to think about. It has been shown that smoking, which also produces AGEs, increases diabetes rates, and it's been shown that AGEs fed to mice increase diabetes rates.

Unfortunately, most of Americans' favorite foods—hamburgers, hot dogs, barbecue, broiled chicken, even Thanksgiving turkey—probably contain a lot of AGEs. If you're already trying to reduce your consumption of saturated and trans fats, high–glycemic index carbohydrates, and highly refined and processed foods, expecting you to give up not only fried hamburgers and steaks but grilled or broiled chicken and fish might seem like the last straw.

As with other dietary recommendations, the answer is not to give up your favorite browned foods altogether but to be aware of their potential dangers. If you have a choice, opt for the food that has the least amount of browning. One piece of barbecue isn't going to give you diabetes. But a lifetime of eating nothing but barbecue could.

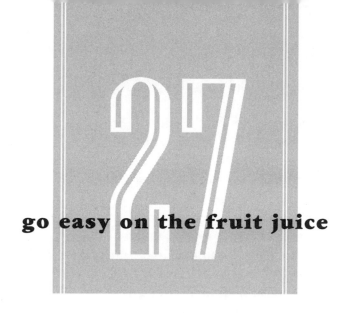

go easy on the fruit juice

RATIONALE:

Although fruits are thought of as healthy foods, fruit juices are often concentrated sources of sugar without any fiber to slow it down.

the current mantra among nutritionists is, "Eat more fruits and vegetables." If interpreted properly, this is good advice. It's much better to eat a bowl of raspberries for dessert than a piece of cheesecake. It's better to have a pear for a snack than a doughnut. And it's clearly better to eat spinach than ice cream.

The problem is that many people associate the word *fruit* with *good,* so anything marketed with the word *fruit* in it may be perceived as a "healthy choice." This is especially true of fruit juices.

Whole fruits do contain sugar (of various kinds, including glucose, fructose, and sucrose in varied proportions), but they also contain a lot of fiber, and as long as you don't have diabetes, the sugar in the fruits shouldn't cause any problems. Many people with diabetes also eat fruit, but they control the amount they eat at one time.

Fruit juices, on the other hand, are loaded with sugar but contain almost no fiber. Liquid foods leave your stomach faster than solid foods, and hence the sugars in juices are dumped into your intestine very fast and quickly make your blood glucose levels go up. People who are having a low blood sugar episode sometimes drink orange juice because it brings their blood glucose level up so fast.

Even worse are "fruit drinks," which may contain a little bit of real fruit juice but consist mostly of flavorings, sometimes including artificial ones, and sweeteners, often high-fructose corn syrup. Because some manufacturers try to attract consumers by labeling such products "low-fat, low-cholesterol," they may appear to be healthy choices. But even more than fruit juices, fruit drinks dump a huge sugar load into your body very quickly. If you have a diabetic tendency, they may overwhelm your pancreas's ability to produce insulin and make your blood glucose levels go above normal.

Does this mean you should never drink fruit juices? Of course not. Fruit juices do contain vitamins and minerals and have some healthy qualities. Just don't overdo it. Be aware that drinking fruit juices is like eating sugar, and when possible, drink real fruit juices instead of fruit drinks.

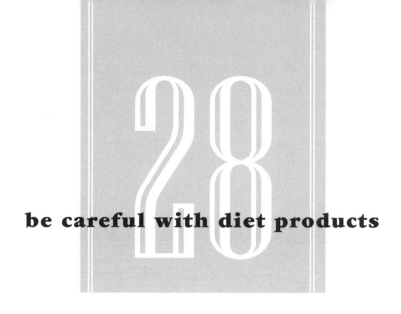

be careful with diet products

in the recent past, America has been going through a fat-phobic phase in which the mantra "fat makes you fat" has become the byword. There is some truth to that mantra. Because fats contain nine calories per gram and carbohydrates and proteins contain only four calories per gram, you can eat a greater weight of carbohydrate and protein and get fewer calories than if you ate the same amount of fat.

There is evidence that *saturated* fat increases insulin resistance, and increased insulin resistance can result in diabetes. Results of studies relating total fat intake to diabetes rates have produced different results. Some show that eating more fat increases diabetes rates. As noted in Tip 6, the Harvard Nurses Study showed no relationship between total fat intake and diabetes rates. But they did find that trans fats increased diabetes rates and unsaturated fats decreased diabetes rates. Thus, trying to avoid saturated fat—as well as trans fats—is probably a good idea.

Today, most "diet" products are low-fat products. In order to capture the ever-increasing market of low-fat dieters, manufacturers have produced more and more low-fat or fat-free "lite" versions of the most popular foods. The problem is, when you remove the fat from a product, you have to substitute something else. Protein is expensive. The cheapest fillers are carbohydrates.

Furthermore, food doesn't taste as good or have such a pleasant "mouth feel" when it has no fat. Hence the manufacturers must seduce the consumer by adding back something to replace the lost taste and mouth feel. That something is often sugar. They hope that the extra sweetness will fool you into not noticing the lack of fat.

Compare the nutrition labels on some full-fat ice cream, some "lite" ice cream, and some frozen yogurt. You'll see that as the fat content goes down, the sugar content usually goes up. The frozen yogurt, although much better in terms of the fat level, usually has more sugar than than the full-fat ice cream.

As with fruit juices, if you have a diabetic tendency, although you don't need to avoid sugar altogether, it's not a good idea to overdose on it.

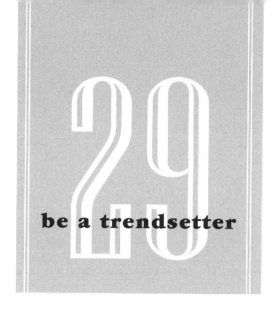

be a trendsetter

RATIONALE:

Type 2 diabetes is becoming epidemic.
If you want to avoid it, you need to be a trendsetter
rather than following the crowd.

the trend in this country is to eat larger and larger amounts of richer and richer food and to let machines do more of the work. Thus if you follow the crowd, you're just increasing your chances of developing diabetes along with everyone else. Instead, you need to be a trendsetter.

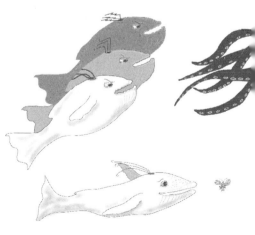

Be different. Eat less food, eat more nutritious food, and move more in your daily activities. When your friends and relatives notice how much better you look and how much more energy you have, they may follow your lead.

It's not always easy to be a trendsetter. Especially when you're young and you want to be just like everyone else, it's hard to order a small chicken salad at a fast-food restaurant if everyone else is getting the Giganto Cheeseburger Deal with a bushel of fries and a gallon of soda. Sometimes it's hard to stand out when you want to melt into the crowd.

But if you want to reduce your chances of getting diabetes, that's the sort of thing you're going to have to learn do. The trick is to make those healthy choices with the confidence of someone who knows what's what, someone who's bored with Giganto Cheeseburgers and wants to move on, to try something different for a change.

If you feel embarrassed about eating different food or walking home when everyone else is catching a bus, if you see those actions as being forced on you by doctor's orders, if you feel deprived because you can't have what all those thin people can have, your peers will sense your embarrassment, and they'll make you feel even worse than you did before. On the other hand, if you adopt a superior air and imply that your peers are all slobs while you're eating healthy food and getting healthy exercise, they're apt to feel threatened and try to make fun of you to save their own egos. Being a successful trendsetter is difficult; you have to develop confidence without appearing superior. Getting a buddy who is also willing to try new foods and new ways of moving helps a lot here (see Tip 36).

If you take charge of your life and make those choices because *you* want to make them, if you learn about new healthier foods that your family and friends haven't tried before, if you think of yourself not as a deprived failure but as a trendsetting gourmet who is going to slowly and non-threateningly show your peers that there's a better way to do things, then your friends may start imitating *you*.

If you're older, you've probably had more experience with standing out from the crowd, but older people get in ruts too. Maybe your Saturday night gang always serves pizza and ice cream before the weekly card game. Shake them up a bit when it's your turn to host. Serve an exotic low-calorie dish—make sure it's especially tasty as well—instead. Maybe they'll be jealous of your creativity and try something similar themselves.

Think of yourself as a pioneer. Learning to lead the pack instead of following in both food choices and ways of moving more means that you're not only improving your own health but you're contributing to the health of your friends. Go for it.

30

eat something red, green, or orange with every meal

RATIONALE:

Brightly colored foods contain antioxidants as well as cancer-preventing compounds. People with diabetes tend to be low in antioxidants.

some people think that vegetables may be one secret of good health. Vegetables contain a lot of vitamins and minerals, but that's not all. Vegetables are chockablock full of beneficial chemicals called *phytochemicals*—which is just a fancy word for "chemicals found in plants"—such as beta-carotein, lutein, and lycopene.

Some vegetables, like members of the *cruciferous* family (broccoli, cauliflower, cabbage, turnip), contain compounds that seem to protect against some cancers.

The highly colored vegetables also contain *antioxidants.* What are antioxidants? Well, sometimes, during all the thousands of chemical reactions that are going on in your body all the time, you produce compounds called *free radicals.* Free radicals are very reactive and when they come in contact with other molecules can damage them and produce even more free radicals.

When free radicals damage your genetic material (DNA), they can cause mutations, including cancerous mutations. When free radicals damage the fats in your body, the damaged fats are much more likely to contribute to *plaques* in your arteries, the lesions that cause *atherosclerosis,* or clogging of your arteries, which can lead to heart attacks. When free radicals damage your skin, they cause wrinkles.

Antioxidants neutralize the free radicals and help prevent all these damaging things.

"Well," you may be thinking, "this is all very interesting. But what the heck does it have to do with diabetes?"

It turns out that people with type 2 diabetes have smaller amounts of antioxidants in their body than people without diabetes. Does the diabetes cause the low levels of antioxidants? Or do the low levels of antioxidants cause diabetes? No one knows for sure.

Just in case it's the latter, that having low levels of antioxidants could contribute to type 2 diabetes, it's certainly a good idea to make sure you get enough. Of course you could choose simply to gulp down a mess of antioxidant pills, which are widely available. But it's not certain that the pills are as effective as the antioxidants you get from food.

You recall the study of beta-carotene that showed that people taking beta-carotene supplements actually had higher lung cancer rates, whereas people getting extra beta-carotene in their food had lower cancer rates. Foods contain a large variety of chemicals, some of which may work together in ways that we do not yet understand. People living in non-Westernized societies in which diabetes is rare are certainly not downing large doses of antioxidants from bottles. They get their vitamins and minerals from their food.

Unfortunately, vegetables are usually more expensive than

eat something red, green, or orange with every meal

starches, so when the budget is tight, it's tempting to serve mashed potatoes instead of spinach, macaroni instead of carrots. But if you possibly can, try to include a colored vegetable or fruit with every meal.

You may not want to eat collard greens or yams with breakfast. But you could have some berries. Berries contain a lot of soluble fiber, which helps slow down your digestion and make your meal last longer, they're not particularly high in calories, and they contain a lot of antioxidants as well. If berries are out of the question, eat an orange. Orange juice is OK, and a lot quicker. But it lacks the beneficial fiber that you get in an orange.

One study did show that people who eat salad vegetables year-round have lower rates of type 2 diabetes. But even if it turns out that eating a lot of antioxidants has nothing to do with your risk of type 2 diabetes, you'll be healthier if you eat a lot of colored vegetables and fruits.

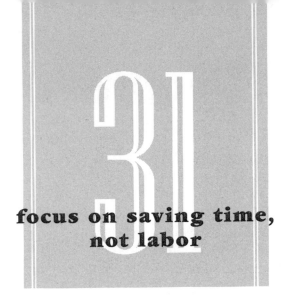

focus on saving time, not labor

R A T I O N A L E :

Labor-saving devices simply reduce the amount of exercise you get in your daily living. Sometimes the old-fashioned way may be better.

if you're living a life of unrelenting toil, for example, walking ten miles every day just to get water to drink or plowing a field without the aid of animals, a few labor-saving devices such as bicycles and tractors would certainly be a blessing.

But most of us today are not living lives of unrelenting toil, despite teenagers' claims to the contrary. In fact, most of us have it pretty easy in that department. I know someone who bought an electric coffee cup that has a little stirring device in the bottom so you can stir up your sugar and milk with less effort. Now, I'd never felt that stirring my coffee was a particularly challenging task, and if there are people who feel that way, no wonder Americans are putting on weight.

Think of all the little chores that people used to do by hand and that we now routinely do with the aid of machines. Just to prepare breakfast, an old-time cook might first carry in some wood to start the wood cookstove, then go to the pump and pump water by hand, carry it into the house, then grind the coffee in a hand mill, then whip up some pancakes or biscuits, beating them a hundred or so strokes by hand, churn some butter (I'm assuming someone else milked the cow), gather eggs from the henhouse, and then cook all this stuff and clean up the dishes by hand—after pumping and carrying more water and heating it up on the woodstove.

Each one of these small chores wouldn't burn that many calories, but an hour spent doing these chores would burn about as many calories as an hour spent walking on a treadmill. And most people in past centuries did similar chores all day long.

I'm not suggesting that everyone return to the days of yore. Besides, your condo might not take well to your suggestion of keeping a cow in the front lobby. But when you're looking at some new wonder "labor-saving" device, you might ask yourself if you really need it.

Most of us *do* need some of the gizmos that our great-great-grandparents didn't have because we simply don't have the time to do everything by hand. But sometimes a labor-saving device might simply be that, something that saves effort. It might not actually save you time.

For example, snowblowers can be great aids if you've got a tremendous driveway to shovel. But equipment like that can sometimes be balky and require a lot of time and effort to start up. Do you really need it? How much time have you spent trying to start a finicky machine or tinkering with it or taking it to the shop? Might a shovel turn out to use less of your time in the long run?

The same is true of a lawn mower. If you live on a huge estate, a power mower makes sense. But if you have a small yard, might an old-fashioned hand mower work just as well and give you some extra exercise at the same time? If you spend thirty minutes on a riding lawn mower, then if you're trying to get thirty minutes of exercise a day, you'll have to spend an additional thirty minutes walking or working out at a gym. If you get thirty minutes of good exercise mowing the lawn by hand, then you'll have an extra thirty minutes to do something you really enjoy. You will also have saved the expense of the big motorized mower and the gas to keep it going, not to mention reducing pollution, so you'll have extra cash to spend on things you enjoy.

Think about it every time you consider purchasing a new labor-saving device. Think about it every time you consider using one you already own. Could I sell this or donate it to a good cause and do the job by hand? Might it be faster by hand? Can I get good exercise if I do it by hand? If the answer is yes, don't worry what the neighbors are doing. Do it your own way.

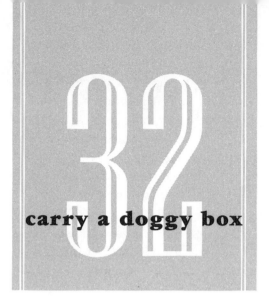

carry a doggy box

R A T I O N A L E :

The best way to deal with gargantuan portions in restaurants is to remove the extra food *before* you start to eat.

except for very upscale restaurants that serve microscopic portions beautifully designed and arranged on your plate, the current trend in American restaurants is to serve bigger and bigger portions. Fast-food joints have been "supersizing" their portions for some time, but even regular restaurants now seem to assume that all their patrons are lumberjacks just in from the timberland.

This strategy seems to work. People tend to gravitate to the place that gives the most, even if it costs more money. And once you become accustomed to huge mounds on your plate, anything else starts to look skimpy.

I don't think we can reform the restaurant business overnight, so what can you do when you're trying to eat reasonable amounts of food? One solution is to just eat what you want and leave the rest. But that's difficult for those of us who can't stand to waste. Another solution is to ask for a doggy bag, which is accepted at most restaurants these days. The problem with that is that it's still tempting to eat more than you want when it's sitting there on your plate.

What I think works the best is to carry your own "doggy box" with you when you eat in restaurants. By a *doggy box,* I mean one of those plastic containers that have compartments for several different foods and also have a very tight fitting lid. If you carry a knapsack, you can keep it there in case you need it. Otherwise you can find a convenient small tote bag to hold the box.

The trick is to put half your meal in the doggy box *before you start to eat.* That way you won't be tempted to eat more than you really want just because the food is there. I don't know if I'm just weird or if other people feel this way, but I've always enjoyed scraping the last bit of food from a plate or an ice cream bowl, or slurping out the last few drops in a milk shake glass (now that I'm adult, I try to do it quietly). It's impossible for me to eat half a yogurt and leave the rest. I need to scrape the container clean. So when I'm eating yogurt, for example, I now scoop out a quarter of a cup into a dish. Then I get the satisfaction of scraping the dish without the temptation to eat too much. When you leave part of your meal on your plate and ask for a doggy bag, you don't get the pleasure of scraping the last bits from the plate.

Here's an extra bonus of the doggy box method: You've got a second meal all ready to heat and serve. If you live alone, you can take the box home and have it for dinner. If you don't like eating the same meal twice in a row, you can put it into the freezer and have it later. If you're going to take lunch to work the next day, it's all ready for you to grab in the morning. Maybe you can even get an extra ten minutes of sleep.

carry a doggy box

In fact, you can use the same method at home if you'd like to lose a little weight but your family insists on the same food you've always had and it's too much trouble to fix you special diet food. Just serve yourself exactly the same amount that you've always eaten, but put some of the food into your doggy box. Voilá. You've just reduced your calorie intake and prepared a snack or tomorrow's lunch all at once. Ideally, you won't be ravenous as a result, just not as stuffed as you used to be (see Tip 41).

If having less food doesn't fill you up, add a high-fiber food to every menu so you can fill up on that. For example, if tonight's dinner is macaroni and cheese with green beans on the side, make sure there are extra green beans so you can have seconds on those.

There's a second bonus of this method: If you eat out a lot, you're cutting your food bills almost in half. If you use the doggy box method, you could calculate how much money you're saving by getting two meals for one. Put the money into a special bank account, and when you've got enough, do something special with it.

Here's another idea that might motivate you to stick to eating smaller portions of overabundant meals. Carry a second change purse with you, and whenever you choose a smaller portion size or decide not to have a doughnut, put the money you've saved into the special change purse. Then send it to a charity that feeds starving children. This way you'll know that you're not only helping yourself become healthier but you're helping to save someone else's life.

You can also use some of the money you've saved to buy better, tastier food, for example some filet mignon instead of hamburger, or raspberries out of season, fresh fish from the expensive fish store, or whatever appeals to you.

Sometimes, eating less can mean eating better.

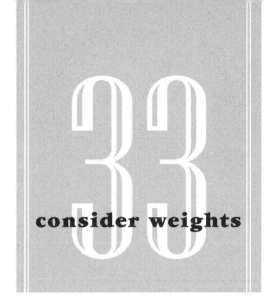

consider weights

RATIONALE:

Lifting weights increases your muscle mass, and it's
muscle that takes the most glucose out of the blood
and burns the most calories.

some people think of weight lifting as something only people who aspire to look like Charles Atlas (or his
bulked-up sister Carlotta) and want to grease up their bulging
muscles would consider doing. Actually, studies have shown
that even people in their nineties can increase their muscle
mass with the regular use of weights.

When people think of exercise, many think of walking and
running or stair-stepping or aerobics classes. This type of exercise is called *aerobic* because it requires a lot of oxygen. It
would be impossible to run a mile while holding your breath.
Aerobic exercise is good to strengthen your heart and lungs.

Weight lifting is called *anaerobic* because it is done for
short periods of time and doesn't require oxygen. You can lift

a weight while holding your breath (although it's better if you don't). Anaerobic exercise isn't as good for your heart and lungs, but it builds muscle mass faster than aerobic exercise.

You may be thinking, "So what. I don't want big muscles, just a little less fat." But increasing your muscle mass is the best thing you can do to lose weight, and also to help keep diabetes at bay. Muscles need more energy than fat, even when you're just sitting around. This is one reason men often find it easier to lose weight than women: Men have a larger ratio of muscle to fat.

Increasing your muscle mass means you'll burn more calories per day, which means you'll lose weight faster eating the same amount of food. If you're lifting weights and you don't lose weight at first, keep in mind that muscle weighs more than fat. You may be losing inches without losing weight as you convert your fat into muscle. And losing fat is your real goal.

Weight lifting also reduces your insulin resistance, and you remember that insulin resistance is a major cause of type 2 diabetes. Insulin resistance depends in part on the ratio of muscle to fat, so the more muscle and the less fat you have, the better. Exercise also increases the amount of fat you burn for energy and thus has a doubly beneficial effect: It reduces your fat and increases your muscle. Muscle is also the main body organ that takes glucose out of the blood. So if you eat a lot of carbohydrates and your blood glucose level goes a little high, having more muscle helps your body get your blood glucose level back to normal quickly.

You can even take advantage of your own body weight to exercise your calf muscles in spare moments when you're standing around waiting for something—or someone. Hold on to something and slowly rise up onto your tiptoes. Stand there for a few seconds and then slowly come down again. Repeat this eight or ten times, or as many times as you can before the bus comes or the water boils or your friend finally shows up. When you gain strength, you can try it without holding on to anything. Then try it standing on just one leg. This exercise should improve your balance, and you may appreciate the fact that it will make your calves more shapely.

For some people, weight lifting can be a bit dull. This is the type of activity that works well with books on tape or your favorite music CDs.

Note: Weight lifting does increase your blood pressure, and if you have high blood pressure you should not lift weights without first checking with your doctor.

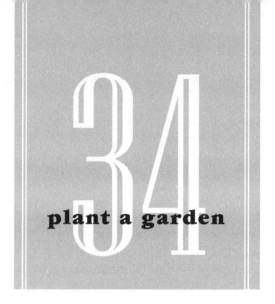

plant a garden

Gardening is both good exercise and a good way to get
healthy, low-cost organic vegetables.

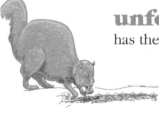

unfortunately, not everyone
has the option of planting a vegetable garden.
If you live in a city high-rise, there's
not a lot of gardening space. But you
don't need forty acres to have a garden. Even if you have a small yard, or
only a terrace or windowsill, you may be able to find a cor-
ner where you could plant at least a few things—some greens
and maybe a tomato or two.

Gardening is good exercise, an example of the kind of
moving more that you should try to do. When you're gardening, you're not only using your muscles, but you're doing
something useful, not just jumping up and down or walking

on a treadmill. With a garden you can get exercise and also feed your family, beautify your house with flowers, and even start a new business.

For example, several women who had come to America from a farming village in Southeast Asia and were living an inactive American lifestyle became diabetic, and their doctor told them they needed to get more exercise. He suggested jogging. They found the idea hilarious and decided to rent some space for a garden instead. They started growing unusual Asian vegetables that quickly became popular locally, and their gardens continued to expand. Now they're running a profitable business as well as getting a lot of exercise, and their blood sugar levels have gone down.

If your garden is small, you can plow it up by hand, which will certainly give your muscles a workout. If it's larger, just maneuvering a rototiller back and forth will burn a lot of calories. Then you have to rake it all out.

Shopping for the best plants and seeds means a lot of walking around, and then you have to come home and plant them. If you have predators in your neighborhood, you'll probably need to install a fence, which should provide even more good muscle-building exercise. Then comes the weeding. Hoeing is good exercise. Sitting down and pulling up the weeds doesn't do much for your muscles except for the hands and arms, but it's certainly better than watching TV.

Your garden isn't for exercise alone, however. Your garden will provide you with produce that is not only fresher and freer from pesticides than what you can buy in the store but also usually has a taste that simply can't be beat. I seem to have a brown thumb, but even so, at least two or three types of vegetables usually survive the cutworms, the chipmunks, and the groundhog.

A warm cucumber from my garden is so good it needs no dressing. Lettuce freshly picked and rushed to the table is a different vegetable from the limp stuff you often find at the grocery store. You can pick your zucchini squashes when they're tiny and crunchy and delicious. You can also plant unusual varieties of vegetables that aren't available in the stores.

When your vegetables are fresh and tasty (and almost free), you're apt to eat a lot more of them. By eating a lot of vegetables you're getting more vitamins and minerals and antioxidants. You're also filling up on high-fiber low–glycemic index foods that will help you eat less of the starchy, greasy stuff that keeps you from losing pounds.

If you simply have no room for a garden at your house, see if there are any community gardens nearby. Sometimes a community group will make a large piece of land available to many local gardeners. If there's no such plot available in your neighborhood, consider getting together with neighbors and starting one.

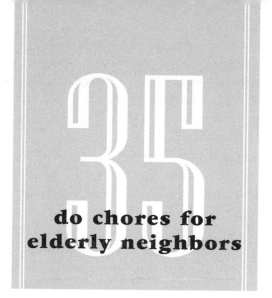

35

do chores for elderly neighbors

R A T I O N A L E :

Any kind of exercise is good, and the idea that you're
helping someone else may help you stick with it.

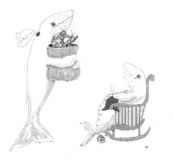

remember that what
you need to do is *move more*, not necessarily exercise more. Anything that
keeps you moving around is beneficial.
What you need is motivation. Do you
have elderly neighbors who are simply
unable to do certain chores themselves? Helping them out
would help you as well.

The best thing would be to explain to them that you need
more exercise and that they'd be doing you a favor if they let
you do some of their chores, especially those that involve
using your muscles. Then they can't refuse out of pride.
They're helping *you*.

Offer to carry out their garbage, mow their lawn, carry heavy groceries into the house for them, move furniture, stack wood, till up a garden space, weed their gardens, walk their dogs, whatever it is that will provide exercise for you and help them in the process.

Do you live in a city neighborhood where it's sometimes dangerous for kids to walk home alone from school? If you're home during the day, you could offer to pick up your neighbor's kids from school and walk home with them, making sure they're safely inside before you say good-bye.

Even better, take them for a walk after school every day, and get them into the habit of being active instead of plopping down in front of the TV when they get home. If they're also at risk for type 2 diabetes—and unfortunately many overweight children today are—you might contribute to their health as well as yours. Now you'll be doing a triple good: helping yourself be more active, helping your neighbor's kids be more active, and helping your neighbors by helping their kids.

Are there nursing homes nearby where there are wheelchair-bound patients who would really love to have someone take them outside? Pushing a wheelchair around for an hour or so would be exercise for you and a real treat for them.

Do you know a library that has books that need reshelving? Offer to help, and don't just stroll slowly down the stacks, but see how quickly (and accurately) you can do the job.

Does your town have a volunteer fire department? What better way to get a little exercise than dragging heavy hoses around. It looks to me as if just carrying all the equipment firefighters wear today would be as much work as lifting weights.

I think you get the general idea here. Look for some kind of volunteer work that involves more physical activity than sitting at endless committee meetings or—even worse—attending fund-raising banquets. Then pledge to do it. It's easy to put off a visit to the gym. It's harder to say no when a neighbor is counting on you.

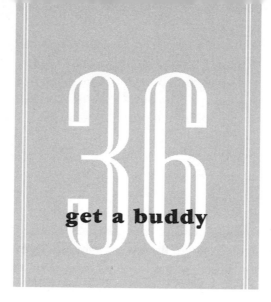

36

get a buddy

RATIONALE:

Knowing you're not alone in your efforts to avoid
diabetes may make those efforts easier.
Besides, it's more fun to do things with friends.

the world is in the midst of a type 2 diabetes epidemic. No one is certain exactly what is causing this explosion of diabetes. Most of the evidence points to increased consumption of calories and decreased expenditure of calories from less physical work. But other factors may be involved as well. Whatever the cause, if you're at risk for diabetes, you're certainly not the only one in your school, your workplace, your neighborhood, or your retirement home.

This means that anything you can do to increase diabetes awareness among your relatives and friends will help. It also means that you should be able to find a diabetes-prevention buddy among your peers, someone who would work together with you to learn more about prevention and to do the things you need to do to reduce your own risks. It's difficult to lobby for better food choices at work or school if you're the only one interested. Get half the group to sign a petition and your chances of success are great.

Find a friend who could also benefit from lifestyle changes and make plans and exchange good recipes and do things together. If you work best when there's a little competition involved, you could view your buddy as a friendly competitor. For example, you could see who could give up smoking the soonest, or who could walk the farthest each week. You can buy a meter to wear all day to count the number of steps you take. Some people even download their results to an Internet site and compete with strangers. Just don't get too compulsive about bettering your buddy. A little competition is good, but too much stress is not. You don't want to exercise so strenuously that you give yourself a heart attack. Use common sense.

If you work best when you have cooperation and support, then your buddy could be there to listen to your latest successes or to commiserate if you've fallen off the wagon. Your buddy would know how difficult it is to stick with lifestyle changes when the life of a couch potato (in your case, a sweet potato of course, as you want to get those colorful vegetables into your life as much as possible) is so much easier, especially after a difficult day at work. And you could celebrate your successes together.

When a lot of people in your neighborhood could benefit from increased exercise, it should be easier to get together and figure out ways to make this possible. For example, lobby for a bicycle trail between your homes and the neighborhood store. If it's not safe to walk in your neighborhood, arrange some kind of security patrol at certain hours, so a group of you can go for a walk.

Some people might have good ideas for adding more fiber to traditional recipes or cooking them with less trans fat. Others might know great places to walk on the weekends. Maybe you could all chip in and buy a treadmill to put in a convenient indoor location that was open to everyone so there would be a safe place to walk when the weather didn't permit walking outdoors.

Instead of complaining about the bottles and cans on the roadside, get a group together and clean up the trash every couple of months. Vermont organizes such a clean-up once a year, called Green Up Day. The walking is good exercise, bending down to pick up trash exercises other muscles, and if your state has deposit bottles and cans, you can donate the profits to the cause of your choice. Of course if you're working busy streets, some kind of safety protection is needed.

Instead of just offering to do a neighbor's chores by yourself, organize a club that does bigger jobs as a group. Paint someone's house (it's probably a good idea to ask first, especially if you paint it bright fuchsia). Build them a new fence. Haul away fallen trees. Get yourselves some snappy uniforms and get some good public relations from the local newspaper. "Diabetes Prevention Team Helps Widow Clean Up from Storm." You'll feel better about yourself and get good exercise at the same time.

If you know teenagers who are at risk, they would benefit from their own separate group. It's hard enough to be a teenager; being a teenager with a disease that limits your ability to eat what your friends eat is a very heavy burden indeed. Anything teens can do to prevent getting diabetes is worth the effort, no matter how unappealing it may seem at the time.

Knowing you're not alone can also help with the depression that may set in when you think how unfair it is that your best friend can eat whatever she wants and never put on an ounce but you may have to control your eating for the rest of your life. Not fair. Of course not. But you're not the only one going through this. Call your buddies and ask them to help you pull through this.

If you can convince a high-risk friend to join you in your efforts, you'll have a double benefit. Having a buddy going through what you're going through will make it more fun. And knowing you've helped someone else help themselves will be a reward all in itself.

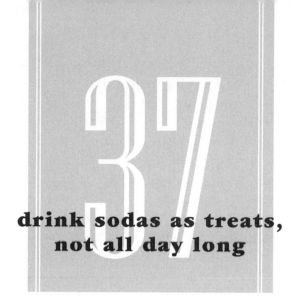

drink sodas as treats, not all day long

RATIONALE:

Sodas contain high levels of fructose that are not found in unprocessed foods. High fructose consumption can increase triglyceride (fat) levels and causes diabetes in rats.

fructose is the name of a sugar that is found in honey and fruit. Small amounts also occur in vegetables. Half of sucrose (table sugar) consists of fructose. The other half is glucose. Eating reasonable amounts of fructose—like eating reasonable amounts of sucrose—is not likely to be harmful.

But in the typical Western diet, fructose has become a major player. Every time you eat sucrose (table sugar), 50 percent of that is fructose. Food manufacturers used to sweeten foods with sucrose. But then they discovered a way to get cheaper sweetening power from corn. This is *high-fructose corn syrup*. Because it's cheaper than cane sugar, it's the preferred sweetener in most manufactured products in America today.

High-fructose corn syrup comes in several different types, the numbers indicating the percentage of fructose in the syrup. HFCS-42 has 42 percent fructose, slightly less fructose than you get from sucrose, and it is also slightly less sweet. It is used in canned fruits when the manufacturers don't want the sweetener to overwhelm the taste of the fruit. HFCS-55 has slightly more fructose than you get from sucrose and is the standard sweetener in soft drinks. HFCS-90, which contains 90 percent fructose and is sweeter than sucrose, is often used in diet or "lite" products when the manufacturers want to distract you from the fact that you're eating less fat by making the product extra sweet.

Thus, except in canned fruits, when you eat products containing high-fructose corn syrup, you're eating even more fructose than you would be if you ate sugar. Eating small amounts should be no problem. But drinking huge amounts of regular soda all day means you're consuming huge amounts of fructose. And because Americans seem to have a "sweet tooth," sweeteners are also added to many processed foods including soups, salad dressings, cold cuts, and sauces. Hence if you drink sodas all day and eat meals that consist primarily of processed foods, you may be taking in a huge amount of fructose every day.

No one knows for certain what eating this much fructose does to your metabolism. Excess fructose can raise the level of triglycerides (fats) in your blood, and high triglyceride levels can contribute to heart disease.

In some animal studies, high levels of fructose increase insulin resistance and are used to make some rodents diabetic. But other studies showed that a high-fructose diet *prevents* diabetes in certain strains of mice. Humans don't always react the same as rodents, so no one knows what a lifetime on a high-fructose diet will do to humans. Do you want to be a guinea pig?

Finally, recall the AGEs (advanced glycation end products), which are formed when glucose reacts with the proteins in your blood. It is thought that AGEs are among the culprits that cause aging and may cause various degenerative diseases like diabetes. Fructose also reacts with proteins. In fact, fructose reacts a lot faster than glucose—ten times or more faster—to form products similar to the AGEs. Thus, eating a lot of fructose could accelerate aging even more than eating table sugar.

Does this mean you should avoid fruit because it contains a lot of fructose? No. The amounts of fructose you'll get from eating these foods is relatively small. Fruit contains beneficial phytochemicals, minerals, and fiber and relatively small amounts of fructose.

But drinking huge supersized glasses of soda with all your meals—not to mention in between—could well overload your system with fructose, and soda has no redeeming values to recommend it.

Then how about diet sodas? Well, the Food and Drug Administration says that the artificial sweeteners used in sodas are safe. But others disagree. Especially if you're young, guzzling huge amounts of these substances is probably not a good idea.

Then what should you do? If possible, *look at sodas as occasional treats, not as your daylong beverage of choice.* Clearly, there *are* times when nothing beats a good cold soda, for example, a hot day when you've worked up a real thirst. There's nothing wrong with the occasional soda in situations like that.

But for general use, try to find a substitute you enjoy. Water is best, but it's not always appealing, especially if you live in a city where the water has been treated with chlorine. Bottled water is better, and if you could afford sodas, you should be able to afford bottled water. Fruit juices are too concentrated in sugar. Beer has problems of its own and promotes excessive weight gain around the middle, the kind of weight gain that contributes to diabetes.

Milk is healthy, but not every adult can tolerate milk. If you can, one study reported in 2002 found that overweight young adults who consumed a lot of dairy foods were less likely to develop insulin resistance—and also less likely to keep increasing weight until they were considered obese—than those who did not. Thus substituting milk for sodas might help reduce your risk of diabetes.

If you avoid highly salted foods—meaning most processed and fast-food meals—and especially if you eat a lot of juicy vegetables, you won't need to drink as many fluids with your meals. The sheep that I raise drink very little water in the summer; they get most of the moisture they need from the grass they eat. You can do the same when you eat lettuce and zucchini and tomatoes and berries.

Try iced tea (unsweetened is best; freshly brewed is better than bottled and also gives you the option of using different kinds of tea). If you really miss the bite from sodas, try drinking plain soda water. Or add a little bit of lemon juice and just a little sweetener of your choice.

You may also want to check the labels of any processed foods you eat and try to reject those that have high-fructose corn syrup as one of the major ingredients, especially the diet products that are apt to contain the 90 percent fructose kind.

You don't have to cut sodas out of your life. But see them as occasional guests, not your daily companions.

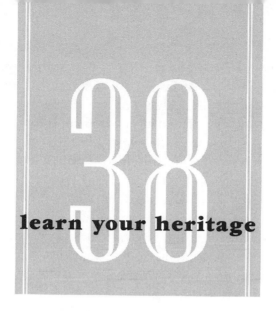

learn your heritage

RATIONALE:

Understanding what variety of type 2 diabetes you're most at risk for will help you take the proper steps to avoid it.

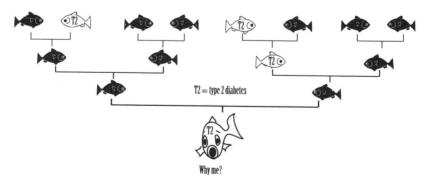

T2 = type 2 diabetes

Why me?

take another look at Figure 2. You can see how complex type 2 diabetes is, because it depends on at least two separate factors: your insulin resistance and the amount of deficiency in your beta cells.

A person with normal beta cells (diabetes threshold A) can have a huge amount of insulin resistance and never develop type 2 diabetes, because the beta cells simply keep churning out more insulin to deal with the insulin resistance. At the other end of the spectrum, a person whose beta cells are able to produce almost no insulin (diabetes threshold D) will develop diabetes even with no insulin resistance at all. And there are various permutations and combinations of the two different factors.

This means that if you suspect your parents or grandparents had a kind of diabetes that was caused primarily from a lot of insulin resistance stemming from being overweight, it's especially important for you to lose weight if you're now overweight, or to keep from gaining weight if you're now at a normal weight.

If your family has always been slim but still developed diabetes, then you should focus on increasing the amount of exercise you get.

For example, let's say your grandfather had a farm and ate fresh fiber-filled food and worked hard all his life. He never got fat but got diabetes at the age of seventy, when he was still milking the cows and doing chores every day. Despite the diabetes, he lived until he was eighty-six. Your father was raised on the farm and grew up getting a lot of exercise, but after college he worked at a desk job at the farm bureau. He was never really fat, but he did put on a few pounds around the middle starting when he was in his midthirties. He got diabetes when he was forty-five. When he was fifty-five he had a major heart attack, and he died several years later.

This family background suggests that simply eating all the right food and getting a lot of exercise may not prevent you from getting diabetes eventually. But exercise should help you postpone the diabetes until you're older. The fewer years you have diabetes, the less likely you are to have complications.

If your mother is still alive, ask if your father changed his eating patterns a lot after he left the farm. If so, what kinds of food did he eat? See if you can see a clear pattern in his off-farm diet. Were there any other differences between his lifestyle and your grandfather's? Did either one smoke? You may not be able to find any definite clues. Sometimes it boils down to chance. But it never hurts to try to find out what it was in your father's lifestyle that may have triggered his diabetes genes.

As another example, let's say your grandfather was a fisherman in Samoa and was lean and fit all his life. He lived until he was eighty and never got diabetes. Your father worked in an office in Honolulu and ate a typical American diet. He was extremely overweight and got diabetes when he was thirty-eight. He's still alive at sixty, but he has some kidney failure and failing eyesight, and his future doesn't look good.

With this kind of a family background, there's a good chance that you can avoid diabetes completely if you are able to keep your weight in the normal range and keep active all your life. That should be a powerful motivation to take charge of your destiny and do whatever it takes to keep slim.

Again, try to find out from family members what kinds of foods your grandfather ate. Your body is probably designed to function well with that kind of diet. If your ancestors ate whales and fish and seals and not a lot of carbohydrate foods, your metabolism may not be designed to process white bread and sugar very well. If your ancestors ate starchy underground vegetables and wild greens and not a lot of meat, your body may not be designed to process fat very well.

If both your parents had diabetes, your risks are *extremely* high. This means you should be especially vigilant and do what you can to keep your weight normal and your activity level high. If, despite all these efforts, you develop diabetes anyway, you should understand that getting diabetes is not a sign of failure on your part. It may just mean that you had an overwhelming genetic tendency to get the disease, especially if both parents were not especially overweight or underactive.

If those in the family who did develop diabetes had a tendency to overeat and avoid moving as much as possible, then the odds are in your favor that by taking action now, you can keep diabetes at bay.

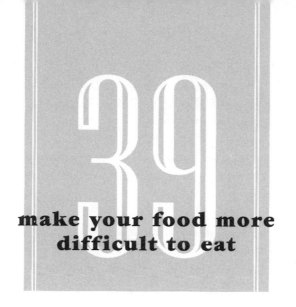

39

make your food more difficult to eat

RATIONALE:

The slower you eat, the more likely you are to feel full before you've eaten too much.

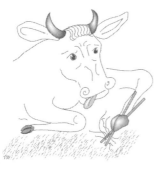

I once knew a woman who hated steak. I asked why. She said because it took too long to cut up and eat. She preferred food that she could shovel in quickly. Yes, she had a weight problem.

When you're hungry and you eat a meal, your hunger will eventually go away. But it takes a while for the "I've had enough" signals to reach your brain, some have estimated about ten to twenty minutes after you start eating. If you eat too quickly, you may have eaten a lot more than you need before those signals get through.

This is one problem with fast food. It's usually not only fast to cook but fast to eat. It doesn't require a lot of peeling or cutting or balancing on a fork. You can pick it up in your hands and gnaw off huge bites at a time.

If you're trying to lose weight, eating quickly is exactly the opposite of what you want to do. Think of yourself not only as a gourmet but as a slow eater. Seek out "slow food" that takes a long time to eat.

See if you can figure out ways to make your food more difficult to eat. For example, unless you're already an expert at using them, try eating with chopsticks. When you use a knife and fork, it's easy to shove a big piece of meat on the fork, cover it with potatoes, and maybe even add some vegetable at the same time. Then you stuff the huge hunk into your mouth all at once. When you use chopsticks, you have to first cut the meal into small bites and then eat one thing at a time.

If you've never used chopsticks before and you're with friends, you can make a game out of it. See who can succeed with the most difficult food. Have a lot of laughs. Laughter helps your digestion as well as slowing down your eating.

Another trick is to eat whole fruits that need to be peeled. Instead of eating pineapple from a can, try buying a whole pineapple and peeling it at the table. Serve fresh mangoes. Or get into the habit of peeling an apple before you eat it. It's not absolutely essential, but unless the apple is organic, it also lowers your exposure to toxic pesticides.

Try buying nuts in their shells. I'm a big fan of raw Brazil nuts, and I could easily eat ten at a time in the blink of an eye. But when I get Brazil nuts in the shells, it's rare that I eat more than two. It's simply too much work. First of all, you practically need a car crusher to get through the thick shells. If I use a strong vice, usually the nut slips out of the vice at the last minute and I end up with twenty-five little pieces of shell all over the floor. Thirty minutes later, when I've retrieved them all, I'm then faced with the task of getting the meat of the nut

make your food more difficult to eat

disengaged from the shell. This usually requires an ice pick. Unfortunately, I can never remember where I put the ice pick, so a fifteen-minute attic to cellar ice pick search ensues. After I've located the ice pick in the dish drainer, I start prying out the nut meat. It certainly tastes delicious, but I usually decide I'd rather do something else for the next hour than attack a second nut.

You get the idea. Think of ways you could make your food more difficult to eat. Grind your coffee beans by hand (you're building arm muscles at the same time). Avoid chopped meats that don't require cutting. Add a little more water to the soup so it takes longer to eat the same number of calories without seriously affecting the taste.

There's one exception to this rule: Make your vegetables easy to eat. That will be an extra enticement to eat more of them.

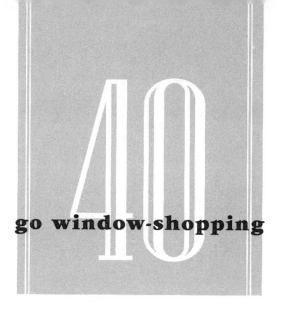

go window-shopping

Any kind of walking is good, so you might as well enjoy it.

you know by now that you want to move more, and to enjoy that increased activity. Walking on a treadmill is good exercise, but it's usually, well, let's face it, not terribly exciting. Why not use your need for more exercise as an excuse to do something you enjoy?

Why not try window-shopping? You could walk briskly for three or four blocks and then move a little slower and look in the windows of interesting stores. Then walk briskly for a few more blocks, and then do some more window-shopping. You could even pick out some things you'd really like to have and plan to reward yourself by buying them when you lose your next ten pounds. If the weather is cold or the downtown stores in your area are not enticing, you can do the same thing in a mall. Just try to avoid the food court. If you live in the suburbs, use your need for exercise as a good excuse to take a trip to a nearby big city to take in the holiday decorations and great window displays in December, or the zoo in the summer, or the shops at any time of the year.

If there aren't many stores of great interest in your town, try going to a boat show, or a museum, or a home show, or whatever it is that you enjoy doing. Use your need for exercise to get you out of the house and to wherever it is that you'd really like to be. Maybe the stamp show or the amusement park the grandchildren love have entrance fees, and you've always worried about the price. Isn't your health worth a little investment?

Remember that to be beneficial, you don't need to walk for thirty minutes or an hour at a time. You can also walk for ten or twenty minutes three times a day. You could do twenty minutes of window-shopping during your lunch hour and then you'd need to spend less time on your treadmill when you got home. Think of other ways to work walking into your daily routine. Be creative. Make the walking fun.

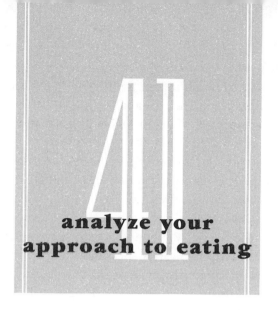

analyze your approach to eating

R A T I O N A L E :

Knowing *why* you eat a lot helps you figure out
how to eat less.

not everyone who is overweight actually eats "a lot." Studies have shown that many overweight people actually eat the same amount as—or even less than—people who are thin. Their bodies just have more efficient ways of dealing with food. Some people call this having "thrifty genes."

Nevertheless, if you want to lose weight—or to keep from gaining more—you need to eat less than you're eating now and to move more than you're moving now, regardless of how little you're currently eating and how much you're currently moving. Understanding why you eat should help you figure out the best strategy that will help you eat less than you do now.

I eat when I'm bored. So for me, the trick is to make sure I'm doing things that interest me (other than eating, that is).

You might eat too much because you are depressed or lonely. Or because you're celebrating good news. Or because people are serving you too much and urging you to "eat up" and clean your plate.

Some people eat too much because they're too polite to say no when someone offers them food. Some can't stand to waste food. Some people eat when it's mealtime, hungry or not. Some people eat when the food looks or smells delicious, hungry or not. In fact, this latter factor is one problem in our current culture. We are surrounded by tempting food—and advertisements urging us to eat even more food—almost all day long.

Faced with all these triggers that make us eat more than we need, it's difficult to cut down. One thing that helps is to figure out what your main triggers are and then to pick a dietary approach that avoids them.

There are several different approaches to eating less. One approach is portion control—eating all the same types of foods, even rich desserts, that you've always eaten, but just in much smaller amounts. One way to do this is to count calories, or some other factor that accomplishes the same thing. This would work well if you were eating too much simply because other people served you portions that were too big.

Let them serve what they like, but just eat less of it. This also works well if you eat in restaurants where the portions are controlled (especially if you carry a doggy box; see Tip 32), but it won't work if you try to fool yourself by taking a huge portion at a buffet so your half-serving will in fact be as large as it always was.

Another approach is to limit the *types* of foods that you eat—for example, limiting fat or limiting carbohydrate or limiting highly refined carbohydrate—but then allowing yourself as much of the remaining foods as you want. This is a good approach if you have trouble limiting portion sizes.

Would you rather eat a quarter cup of premium ice cream or a whole cup of reduced-calorie ice cream or cut ice cream out of your life entirely and eat only fruit instead? Think of these things and choose an eating plan that seems to satisfy your own personal needs. Don't be influenced by what works for your husband, wife, boyfriend, or mother-in-law. Your needs may be different.

You should also analyze your hunger and learn to differentiate *hunger* from *appetite*. There are many levels of hunger, as shown below. The first level is real hunger. Real hunger hurts. I think I've been really hungry only once in my life, when I was young and shy and got stranded in a foreign country where I was afraid to go into a restaurant by myself. Trying to sightsee, I noticed that instead I was gravitating to outdoor cafés and standing around staring at the food on other people's plates. I also had a great pain in my stomach.

The Hunger Pyramid

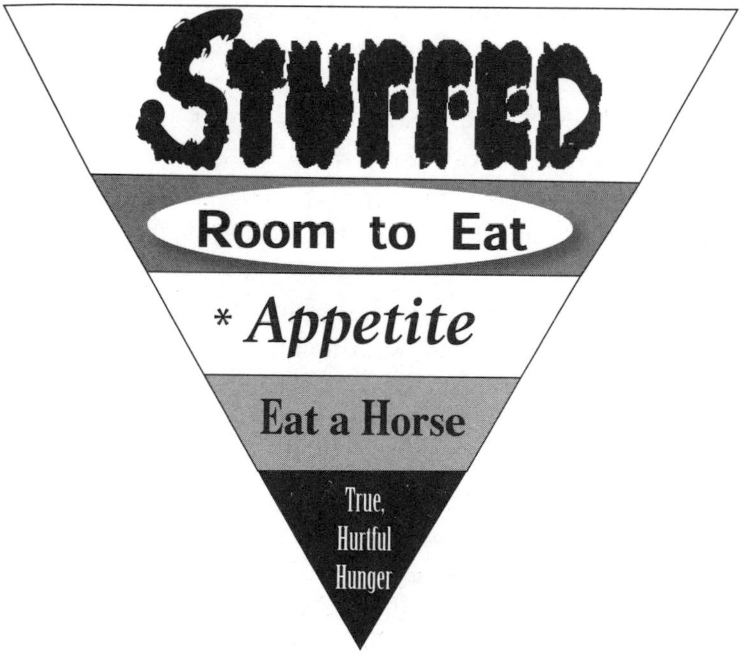

STUFFED

Room to Eat

* Appetite

Eat a Horse

True, Hurtful Hunger

The next level of hunger is what we often call *ravenous hunger*, the kind in which you say you could eat a horse. I'll call this the Eat-a-Horse level. This isn't really true hunger, just a ravenous appetite. It's a good thing to avoid, because when you have a ravenous appetite, you're apt to eat quickly and end up eating more than you really need.

The next level, which I'll call the Appetite level, is simply having a good appetite, looking forward to a meal with pleasure, and truly enjoying every bite because it satisfies your appetite as well as tasting good. This level is a good kind of appetite to have, because it means you haven't overeaten at a previous meal or snack, and it makes everything you eat taste even better: The old saying "Hunger is the best sauce" is certainly true. But you're not so ravenous that you can't eat slowly and savor every bite.

The next level, which I'll call Room to Eat, is not having much appetite at all, just not being stuffed. At this level you're able to eat a meal even if you don't really need to eat. This is the kind of hunger level that leads to unnecessary snacking if you're bored or if someone offers you a tempting treat.

The next level, being so full you can't even eat your favorite dessert, is of course not hunger at all but its opposite: Stuffed.

When you're tempted to eat something, it helps to think about what kind of hunger you have. Do you have a real appetite (Appetite level)? If so, eating something, even just a little, may be a good idea so you can avoid getting into the Eat-a-Horse level, when you'd be more apt to overeat. Or are you just not stuffed (Room-to-Eat level) and you're eating for some reason other than hunger? If so, saying "No thank you" would be a better idea.

Another thing to do is to learn to stop eating when you reach the Room-to-Eat level. When urged to have seconds or thirds, or when I was at an all-you-can-eat buffet, I used to eat until I felt stuffed. That was the signal to stop. It's much bet-

analyze your approach to eating

ter to eat a small portion of various foods and then enjoy the conversation if you're with a group or get up from the table if you're alone. If you still have a really good appetite after fifteen or thirty minutes, you should have some more of the protein or high-fiber parts of the meal. Usually, though, you'll find you've moved into the Room-to-Eat level, even with much less food than you're accustomed to eating. Sure, you *could* eat more if you wanted. But you don't *need* to eat more.

One trick of successful dieting is to learn to understand that the mild appetite of Room to Eat doesn't need feeding. You're not going to starve to death. Having a mild appetite never killed anyone. And it's a lot better than the consequences of constantly feeding that mild appetite, namely, gaining more weight and perhaps developing diabetes.

If you find that you're constantly in the Eat-a-Horse or even the Appetite hunger level no matter how much you eat, there may be something wrong with your appetite control. Consult a physician—perhaps an endocrinologist—about this. There are people who are resistant to normal appetite controls, just as there are people who are resistant to insulin.

Some people who have always had ravenous appetites shortly after eating high-carbohydrate meals find that low-carbohydrate diets help control their hunger and hence help with weight loss. This may be especially true of people who don't have good control of their blood sugar levels and are hence headed toward diabetes.

It takes a while to learn new approaches to eating, and it's difficult when everyone else everywhere you look seems to be eating larger and larger meals more and more often. But it can be done. And if you succeed, you'll have accomplished something you can be proud of.

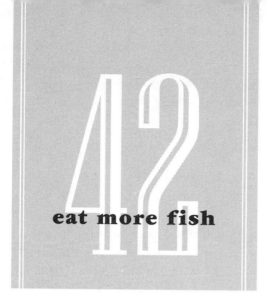

eat more fish

Compounds in fish oils reduce insulin resistance and hence may lower your risk of diabetes.

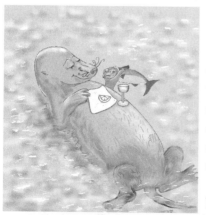

as I outlined in Tip 6, fatty acids can be either saturated or unsaturated. But the saga of fats gets even more complicated than that. It turns out that not all unsaturated fats are created equal.

Unsaturated fatty acids can be divided into two general categories called *omega-3* and *omega-6* (sometimes called n-3 and n-6; it means the same thing). Most vegetable oils contain mostly omega-6. Cold water fish and a very few vegetable products, including flaxseed and purslane, are high in omega-

3 oils, which are otherwise scarce in the typical Western diet.

Each type of fatty acid has opposite effects on various systems in the body. For example, omega-6 oils tend to make the blood clot. Omega-3 oils tend to keep the blood from clotting. You need to have your blood clot or you might bleed to death every time you got a cut. But if your blood clots too easily, you're apt to have serious clots that cause heart attacks. Thus the goal is to keep these two opposing factors in balance.

When people eat diets consisting of wild game and wild plants, their consumption of omega-6 and omega-3 fats is in a ratio of approximately 1:1 or 2:1. Our Western diet, with high consumption of vegetable oils, has a much higher amount of omega-6 and a much lower amount of omega-3, with a ratio that can be as high as 50:1, or fifty times as much omega-6 as omega-3. Some people think this is contributing to our poor health.

A study reported in 2002 found that three months of supplementation with a particular omega-3 component of fish oil—docosahexaenoic acid (DHA)—reduced insulin resistance in overweight people who were insulin resistant. They said the improvement was "clinically significant" in half of the twelve people in the study. Because the number of people in the study was small, the results were only preliminary. But the researchers pointed out that Greenland Eskimos who get a lot of omega-3 fatty acids from eating blubber have very low rates of diabetes.

Thus any chance you have to increase your omega-3 consumption is a good thing. Eating fatty fish like salmon, sardines, mackeral, halibut, or herring is one way to get more omega-3 fatty acids. Just eating two servings a week of cold water fish like these should give you enough omega-3 oils.

If for some reason you can't eat fish, you can get the oils from fish oil supplements. But it's always better to get your nutrients from real foods. In the past, researchers have found that some fish oil supplements *increase* insulin resistance in some people with diabetes. It may depend on the particular supplement or on how fresh the oils are. Fish oils get rancid fairly easily. Also, concentrated fish oils are "blood thinners," and if you're taking other blood thinners such as aspirin, vitamin E, *Ginkgo biloba,* ginger, garlic, or fenugreek, you should be cautious with fish oils.

A very few plants also contain significant amounts of omega-3 oils, and these include flaxseed and purslane (*Portulaca oleracea*). Purslane is a low-growing succulent plant that many people in this country consider to be a weed, but in India, Iran, and some other countries it is cultivated as a vegetable. It is said to have been one of Mahatma Gandhi's favorite vegetables. You can eat it raw in salads; it adds a slightly sour taste. Or you can cook it as a vegetable.

Because the omega-6 fatty acids are common in our diet, any chance you have to eat more omega-3 fatty acids should improve your health.

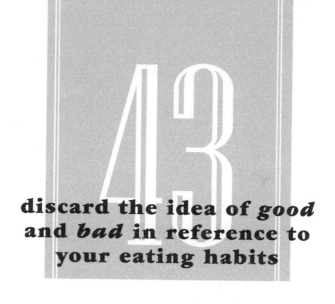

discard the idea of *good* and *bad* in reference to your eating habits

R A T I O N A L E :

The labels *good* and *bad* just make you feel guilty when you give in to temptation and may make you eat more in the long run.

how many times have you said, or heard someone else say, "I was *bad* today. I had cheesecake (or some other "forbidden" food) and ice cream too"? Or "I was a *good boy*. I ate my spinach."

Thinking of yourself as bad when you're human and you give in to temptation and eat something you know you shouldn't just puts you in the position of being a child, someone who has been told what to do and who has disobeyed. If you think of yourself as being bad, you may think of yourself as a failure, a real loser. And if you're a loser, you'll never succeed with your diet, so why bother? Thinking this way means you're just setting yourself up for failure.

Even if you say you're a "good girl" or a "good boy," you're seeing yourself as a powerless person under someone else's control. When you really *were* a child, if Mom said you couldn't have a cookie before dinner, naturally you'd try as hard as possible to sneak one anyway. Rebelling against authority is often a lot of fun.

So if you still see yourself as a powerless pawn under some doctor's or dietician's orders to follow a strict diet, aren't you just going to be more tempted to cheat? "If no one sees me eating this cookie, it won't count."

Instead, think of yourself as a responsible adult who is embarking on a new way of eating not because someone told you that you had to lose fifty pounds but because you *want* to take control of your health.

Remember that no one is perfect. If you were, all your friends would hate you. So even if you've found the perfect way of eating that works for you most of the time, there are going to be times when you eat foods that aren't on your eating plan, or when you eat more than you'd planned to eat.

When this happens, don't think of yourself as "cheating." Don't think of yourself as bad. Think of yourself as someone who just decided that for right now, the benefits of tasting this food or eating a little extra of that food are worth the risks. Sometimes being too strict can just set up cravings that will eventually lead to binging. You're an adult, and you're in charge. You know the difference between a small lapse and throwing your diet to the winds. At your next meal you'll do better. No guilt.

If you do eat something that isn't on your plan, remember that dieting isn't an all-or-nothing thing. If you lapse at lunch, that's no reason to think, "Oh well. I've blown the diet. Might as well pig out for supper. Tomorrow I'll start the diet again, and I'll be *really really* good." That's the kind of thinking that leads to postponing the start of a diet for week after week, even year after year. I know: I've been there, done that, got the T-shirt.

Instead, if you eat a little extra for lunch, try to eat a little less for dinner. That will keep you on track with sensible, steady progress instead of yo-yo dieting in which rapid weight loss is followed by total abandonment and regaining of everything you've worked so hard to lose.

discard the idea of *good* and *bad* in reference to your eating habits

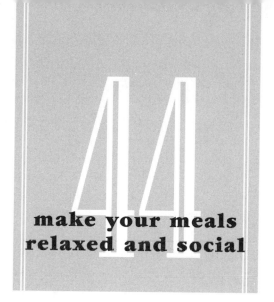

make your meals relaxed and social

R A T I O N A L E :

If meals are relaxed, pleasant times for socializing, you'll
be able to enjoy them even when you're eating less.

one problem with modern American life is
that our meals have become too fast, often eaten on the run
or at a desk. Even when families serve a family dinner, conversation may be hampered by a blaring TV, or teenagers may
gulp their food so they can get away as quickly as possible to
be with their peers.

If you're trying to eat less, there are several traps to this
approach to eating. Food that is designed to be eaten quickly,
even if it's not the burgers and fries that we usually think of
when we refer to *fast food,* is often starchy and overcooked,
so you can gulp it down without having to cut or chew. It's
exactly the opposite kind of food from what you—a budding
gourmet—want to eat. You need food that is a little more difficult to eat, that takes a long time to cut and chew.

When you eat quickly, you are apt to eat more than you need before your natural appetite-suppressing mechanisms kick in. One study showed that ten minutes after twenty-one adults started eating, their urge to eat more decreased. When you eat slowly, you'll tend to eat less without realizing it or feeling deprived.

Another advantage to slower, more social eating, is that once you've had enough, you can focus on the conversation and extend the break from work or your daily routine even when you're not eating any more, instead of quickly eating what you need and going right back to work—or getting right up and doing the dishes. If your table companions are all talking, or singing, or even yelling at each other, you've got a good show to watch, and it's easier to ignore the extra food you shouldn't have. If you feel deprived when everyone else is still eating, order a large cup of coffee or tea, a small glass of wine, or even an extra bowl of soup, so you'll be eating or drinking too while they finish up their abundant portions. Or eat a couple of bites, savoring the flavor and texture of your food, and then focus on the conversation. Then have a few more bites. Then back to the conversation. When you don't try to eat and converse at the same time, you'll both be able to focus on the food that you do eat and spread your meal out over a longer period of time.

Scientists have studied the food patterns of people in the Mediterranean region because Mediterranean people who are maintaining their traditional way of life have very low rates of heart disease. Although traditional lifestyles are changing, the old ways of eating might be a factor. In some places, the main meal of the day was served at noon. Workers went home for the midday meal and sometimes even took a nap before returning to work in the afternoon.

The whole family was there. The meal was often served in many courses, which slowed it down. You might start with soup, and then you'd have a meat dish, and after that you'd have a vegetable dish. Then you might have a salad. And then some fruit. And then some cheese. All this takes time. Between courses, your appetite-suppressing mechanisms would have a chance to kick in. The break from on-the-job stresses would also tend to reduce stress hormone levels.

Such a meal also requires a lot of separate dishes, and as working couples become the norm, it becomes more and more difficult to maintain a lifestyle like that. Today many of you probably have to grab a bite while you work at your desk, or perhaps you live alone and don't have the option of a drawn-out family dinner. But the closer you can come to such an approach to eating, the easier it should be for you to enjoy your mealtimes while eating less food.

There's another factor in Mediterranean eating styles that may help keep diabetes away. Red wine is commonly drunk with meals. Moderate drinking of red wine has been associated with lower rates of diabetes. One study of 41,000 health professionals showed that the moderate drinkers were close to half as likely to develop diabetes as the nondrinkers.

People who drink red wine with their meals also seem to have healthier hearts. This is sometimes referred to as *the French paradox*. It's paradoxical because the traditional French diet is filled with rich sauces oozing with saturated fat, and yet the French have relatively low rates of heart disease. Studies have shown that drinking red wine can increase levels of HDL, the beneficial type of cholesterol that seems to reduce the risk of heart disease. Some studies have suggested that the benefit stems from phytochemicals in the wine and others suggest that it comes from the alcohol itself.

Red wine isn't usually the kind of drink you gulp down in one swallow. It's always possible that populations that drink wine with meals also have more relaxed, stretched-out meals. A little wine might help to reduce stress.

Obviously this does not mean it's a good idea to drink yourself into the gutter every night. The same studies that showed that moderate drinkers (one drink for women or two for men) had lower rates of diabetes showed that heavier drinkers had higher diabetes rates.

All alcohol contains calories. Beer, especially, may contribute to weight gain, including the large "beer belly" (apple shape) that often goes along with a high diabetes risk.

No one should consider taking up drinking to prevent diabetes. But slowing down, enjoying company with your meals, and having a *small* glass of wine as you eat might all help reduce your levels of stress hormones and thus your insulin resistance. And as you know by now, less insulin resistance reduces your chances of developing diabetes.

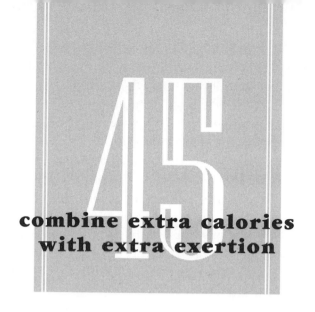

combine extra calories with extra exertion

R A T I O N A L E :

When you know you've eaten more than you should,
you can minimize the damage by adding extra exertion
to your usual routine.

no one is perfect, and sticking to a strict diet for the rest of your life is a herculean task that no one but a saint could do—and I read somewhere that saints have very high rates of cancer, so being a saint apparently isn't very healthy.

There are going to be times when temptation is overwhelming. Once you have diabetes, giving in to temptation may cause immediate harm. Your blood glucose levels will go up, your vision may become blurry, and you may feel fatigue, or even tingling in your arms and legs. But if you're being careful and you've managed to keep diabetes at bay, then the occasional treat or calorie blowout isn't going to ruin your health. It may put your weight loss onto a stall, however.

One way to overcome this is to add exercise to balance out

the increase in calories consumed. Table 3 gives an example of the amounts of calories burned for various types of exercise for a woman weighing 125 pounds and a man weighing 250 pounds. You can see that a heavier person actually burns more calories doing the same amount of work, because simply carrying around all that extra weight requires extra work.

Note that these numbers are simply approximations. Some people may burn more calories and some may burn fewer doing the same amount of work, because everyone's physiology is a little different. But this gives you a general idea.

The trick here is to do the extra exercise *before* you have the extra food. Here's why. If you go out to a special celebration and get tempted by the lemon chiffon cake with the sour cream icing, you may think, "Well, I could have a large piece of that, and then I could do extra weight lifting this evening to work it off." But then when evening comes, you're tired and you think, "Well, I could do the extra work tomorrow." And tomorrow and tomorrow. I know. I've been there. Then you not only don't do the extra exercise, but you feel guilty as well.

If instead you know you're going to a big celebration, you can do the extra work or exercise or play *before* you go. Then you can say to yourself, "Well, I just burned an extra 500 calories. That means I can eat an extra 500 calories at the party. Let's see what I'll pick."

Then you can eat something extra and not feel guilty about it. Just don't do so much extra exertion right before the event that you have a ravenous appetite and end up eating 1000 extra calories instead of 500. As always, use common sense.

TABLE 3

CALORIES BURNED PER HOUR WITH VARIOUS ACTIVITIES

Activity	125-lb woman	250-lb man
Sleeping	51	85
Watching TV	57	95
Computer work or attending meetings	85	142
Office work, desk	102	170
Driving farm machinery, playing catch, pushing a stroller, vacuuming, fishing from a boat, office work while standing, or walking at 2 mph	142	236
Lawn mowing:		
Riding mower	142	236
Power push mower	255	425
Old-fashioned push mower	340	567
Bowling, hobby carpentry, driving a bus or semi, playing regular Frisbee, or nursing	170	284
Walking:		
4 mph	227	378
2 mph	142	246
Shooting baskets, hanging sheetrock, or using a snowblower (walk-behind)	255	425
Painting house or gathering maple sap by hand	283	470
Folkdancing	312	520
General hiking, shoveling snow	340	567
Backpacking or jogging	397	662
Mountain biking	482	804
Jumprope, moderate	567	946
Rock climbing	623	1040
Ice skating, racing	850	1418

Note: These figures come from the Web site *www.caloriesperhour.com*. They were calculated for a woman weighing 125 pounds and a man weighing 250 pounds, both 35 years old and both five feet nine inches tall. Factors that increase calorie use include sex (men burn more calories than women even at the same age, height, and weight), age (younger people burn more calories than older ones), and height (a taller person burns more calories than a shorter person).

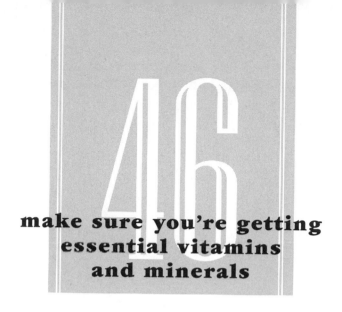

make sure you're getting essential vitamins and minerals

R A T I O N A L E :

Low levels of some vitamins and minerals have been associated with type 2 diabetes.

when you're eating a lot of whole foods including a variety of vegetables and fruits grown in soil that contains the proper nutrients, you're probably getting all the vitamins and minerals you need for good health. But when you're eating a lot of processed foods—even foods "fortified" with certain vitamins and minerals—you may not be getting enough vitamins and minerals from your food. A lack of some of these substances has been associated with type 2 diabetes risk.

For example, it is known that a deficiency of the minerals chromium and vanadium can cause type 2 diabetes. One study in China, where chromium deficiencies were shown to exist, showed that supplementing the diet with chromium reduced the incidence of type 2 diabetes.

Some people say that most Americans are not deficient in chromium, which is needed for the body to process glucose. However, when you eat a lot of refined carbohydrates, you're not getting chromium in these foods. Furthermore, the chromium that you have may be depleted in the process of digesting the carbohydrates. Thus your chromium levels may gradually get lower and lower.

Other vitamins and minerals that have been reported to be associated with diabetes include magnesium, zinc, and vitamin D.

If X is *associated with* Y it does not always mean that X *causes* Y. In some cases, a deficiency of some nutrient might be caused by diabetes genes rather than causing the diabetic tendency. However, just in case deficiencies do help cause type 2 diabetes, it's a good idea to be cautious. Eating vegetables is the best way to get your vitamins and minerals. But if for some reason you simply can't eat anything but bread and cereal, you should make sure you're getting enough vitamins and minerals with a multipurpose vitamin pill.

It costs a little extra, but it's a lot cheaper than dealing with diabetes.

47

spend more time with little children

RATIONALE:

Little children are balls of energy, and just following them around will help keep you active.

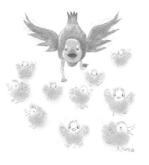

I once read about a trained athlete who was assigned to follow a two-year-old child around all day and do exactly the same things that the child did. By the end of the day, the athlete was bushed.

The story may not be true, but it could be. Little children never seem to sit still. Why walk when you can run? Even if you're not trying to imitate their every move, just being around little children seems to rev up the metabolism a bit.

If you have little children of your own, you may think that what you really need is some quiet time to yourself instead of more time with the perpetual motion machines that are your kids. Maybe you could figure out some kind of activity that would be fun for them while providing good exercise for you.

So what if the lawn needs mowing and the windows need washing. Let the lawn get a quarter inch higher and live with the smudge on the window. Take the kids to the zoo or to the park instead, where you'll do a lot of walking and the kids will have a lot of fun. Or show them how to throw a football, join them in tag, show them how you used to play hopscotch or jump rope, or teach them how to kick a soccer ball.

Invite your grandchildren over for the day, and make sure you do active things together. Or take on some daytime babysitting jobs and join the kids in their active games or take them for a hike. You'll be much more popular than the babysitter who plops the kids in front of the TV and reads movie magazines all day.

Remember, you want to move more. It doesn't matter what you do to increase your movement. It makes a lot more sense to enjoy active things with your children—or grandchildren or younger friends—than to ignore them so you can spend hours at a gym.

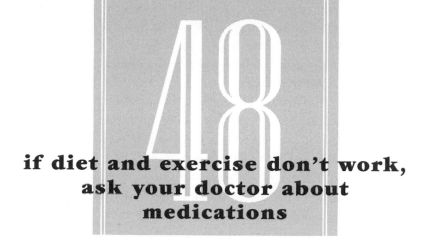

if diet and exercise don't work, ask your doctor about medications

RATIONALE:

New research is finding drugs that may help reduce the risk of diabetes.

the best approach to trying to reduce your diabetes risk—especially if you are young—is to work hard to ensure that you will never become overweight, or to lose weight if you are already above your ideal weight, and to remain active throughout your life. If you're young, you probably won't want to start on a medication that you'll have to take for the rest of your life. All medications have side effects, and the longer you take a medication, the greater the chance that it will cause some harm.

On the other hand, we *know* that diabetes will cause harm, and the longer you have diabetes, the greater the probability that the complications of the disease will be serious.

Thus if you've tried your best at eating less and moving more and they haven't produced the results you want, you might want to discuss with your doctor the possibility of trying some drugs that have been shown to reduce the risk of diabetes.

The Diabetes Prevention Program that I mentioned earlier showed that diet and exercise reduced by 58 percent the number of people who progressed from prediabetes to full-blown diabetes. One drug, metformin, also reduced the diabetes rate, but only by 31 percent, not as much as the diet and exercise did. Thus if for some reason you're not able to exercise, or if you simply can't lose weight even when you cut way back on your calories, you might think about trying metformin, which has several effects, one of which is to reduce insulin resistance. Some people also find that it's easier to lose weight when they're on metformin, because it tends to reduce the appetite. Others find that it causes nausea and diarrhea and they can't tolerate the drug.

Two other types of drug called *ACE* (angiotensin-converting enzyme) *inhibitors* and the related angiotensin II receptor blockers (*ARBs*) are usually used to reduce blood pressure. In one trial, researchers found that an ACE inhibitor helped reduce complications in people who already had diabetes. They were expecting this. But to the surprise of the researchers, the ACE inhibitor also reduced the number of people who progressed to diabetes during the trial. In another study, an ARB did the same thing.

ACE inhibitors and ARBs have not yet been approved for preventive therapy, but they could be in the future.

One study also showed that a drug in the *statin* class was associated with lower rates of diabetes. Others showed that a drug called *acarbose* that reduces blood glucose levels and a drug in the *glitazone* class that reduces insulin resistance reduced diabetes rates in people at high risk. As time passes, other drugs may also be shown to be useful in preventing diabetes. So it's a good idea to keep in touch with your doctor to stay informed about this.

If you think you might be at risk for diabetes but don't really have a regular doctor, it might be a good idea to look around now, *before* you have a real problem, to try to find a doctor you like and can work with. Especially if you're overweight, you may have had bad experiences with medical people in the past. Maybe they blamed all your medical problems on your weight. Maybe they even put you down or made fun of you because of your excess weight.

Don't lose hope. There *are* sensitive doctors who do understand the problems of people who gain weight easily and have problems getting it off again. Also, attitudes about overweight people are beginning to change. Some doctors have admitted that in the past physicians tended to blame patients for being overweight, but as new facts about appetite-controlling hormones are being discovered, they are realizing that many factors are involved.

If you're in an HMO, or if you see doctors at a clinic, you might not have a lot of choice. But if you can, ask around and see if you can find a doctor you like. If you establish a good relationship with a doctor now, *before* you get diabetes, the doctor may be able to help you make the changes you need to make to ensure that you *never* get the disease.

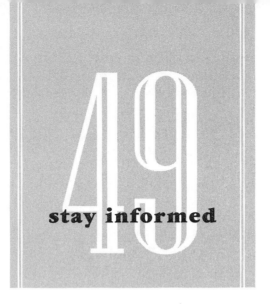

49

stay informed

RATIONALE:

Staying informed about the latest findings may help you avoid getting the disease.

diabetes information is exploding almost as fast as the rates of type 2 diabetes. Sometimes it seems as if every day a new report comes out blaming this factor or that factor for the sudden increase in the rates of type 2 diabetes in this country.

The same is true of treatments for diabetes, and eventually some of the drugs developed to treat diabetes may turn out to be useful for prevention as well. Metformin is one drug that appears promising in this area.

Nutritional theories are also rapidly changing as new information becomes available. For example, in the 1950s, people were told to avoid "starchy" foods such as pasta and potatoes if they wanted to avoid getting fat. Then in the 1970s and

1980s, fat became the villain, and the public was urged to "get the fat out" and to eat "complex carbohydrates" like pasta and potatoes instead. The Food and Drug Administration published a Food Pyramid that suggested that people emphasize complex carbohydrates in their diet, showing pictures of flour, bread, rice, and potatoes as examples.

Now, with information about the glycemic index and the glycemic load becoming more well known, the pendulum is turning the other way. It turns out that white flour, white bread, white rice, and potatoes have high glycemic index values and may be contributing to high blood glucose levels after meals, which could lead to insulin resistance and type 2 diabetes.

The same is true of fat. First all fat was bad. Then saturated fat was supposed to be bad but unsaturated fat was supposed to be good. Then it turned out there were different kinds of unsaturated fats, some of which were oxidized very quickly and caused damage to the body and others of which formed trans fats under certain conditions. Today monounsaturated fats are supposed to be good. Who knows what tomorrow will bring.

The best way to deal with all of this is, first, not to take any news report of the latest nutritional finding as the last word. Listen to the new findings. Keep them in your head. But don't go overboard. For example, if you understand that most Americans eat too many omega-6 fatty acids and don't eat enough omega-3 fatty acids, don't stop eating omega-6 fatty acids altogether while consuming huge amounts of mackerel and flaxseed and taking fish oil supplements as well. You might end up with the opposite problem: too many omega-3 and not enough omega-6 fatty acids. The important thing is to keep them in balance, and the best way to keep them in balance is to eat real foods.

The second way to deal with this is to stay informed. Our ideas of what is healthy will naturally change as new information comes to light. Even highly trained nutritionists can't make good judgments before they have the facts. The information in this book should give you a start, but it is necessarily brief. My book *The First Year—Type 2 Diabetes* goes into more detail about the composition of food and how it affects blood glucose levels. Basic books on nutrition will tell you more. News and magazine articles will keep you informed of the latest developments on nutrition, exercise, and type 2 diabetes risks.

If you have access to the Internet—and most people can reach the Internet through their local library if not at home—you can find a lot of information there. There is also a lot of misleading information on the Internet, as well as snake-oil salesmen, and you need to learn how to sift the good from the bad. This is not an impossible task. Most people can differentiate information found in a cheap tabloid from that found in *Scientific American*. The Internet is the same. Check the source of any information before you take it too seriously. If it seems too good to be true ("Lose 100 pounds in one week with no dieting"), it probably is.

Information is your best weapon against type 2 diabetes.

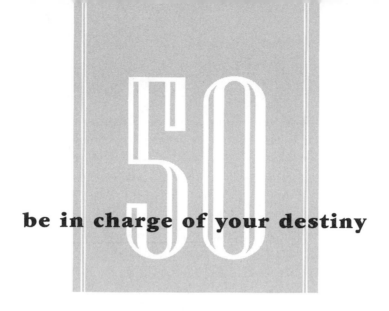

be in charge of your destiny

RATIONALE:

It's your health that is involved, and you're more apt to succeed in making beneficial changes in your lifestyle if you're in the driver's seat.

if you want to avoid diabetes—and who doesn't?— you can ask your doctor or a nurse or even a friend to help you in your efforts. But in the long haul, you are the only one who can make the changes that will reduce your risk of getting diabetes.

Sure, your doctor or a dietician can prescribe a diet for you. But unless you decide to follow that diet—or find another one that you like better, or decide not to follow a diet at all but to become a gourmet who eats small portions of delicious-tasting food—it's not going to do any good. Someone can tell you that it would be a good idea for you to get more exercise, but unless you decide yourself that it's something you want to do, you're not going to do it.

Everyone's a little different, of course. I'm sort of a contrarian myself. If my doctor told me to lose five pounds, I'd probably gain ten pounds just to prove that no one can boss me around. If you've been overweight all your life, you may have been humiliated by health care people who suggested that you're overweight because you have no willpower and you're too lazy to exercise. If so, you may not be apt to want to try yet another campaign to try to turn yourself into a sleek sylph who will attract men from miles away or a muscular athlete who will get all the girls in the end.

Just remember that it's your health that is at stake here. Don't try to move your muscles more because some doctor or some guy on TV or some article in a health journal—or even this book—told you that you should. Try to move your muscles more because *you want to take control of your health*. Put your destiny in your own hands. Make up your mind that you can succeed at this. You can reduce your risks of diabetes—and other ailments as well.

If you're overweight, try to lose weight. But if nothing works, even when you're trying your best, don't despair. Focus on exercising your muscles more. Find something active that you enjoy doing. And do it. Not because you're supposed to. But because you want to.

It's *your health* we're talking about here. Depriving yourself of the rich treats your skinny friends are having is no fun. But having diabetes is no fun either. You're lucky. You don't have diabetes yet. You may be able to keep it at a distance for many years to come.

Don't wait. Do something now, before it's too late. Take charge. Remember the mantra: Eat less and move more. Eat less and move more. Don't worry about what other people say, or other people do. You're the important one here. You have power over your own health. Take that power and use it.

AFTERWORD

as you should understand by now, the cause of type 2 diabetes is complex and not completely understood. Some people may do all the right things to prevent it and still come down with the disease. If this happens to you, don't blame yourself.

Take another look at Figure 2, which is actually a simplification of the real-world situation. You can see that even this simplified version of the cause of type 2 diabetes is complex. Joe might have a lot of insulin resistance and just a little beta cell failure. Jolene might have a lot of beta cell failure and just a little insulin resistance. All kinds of other combinations are possible.

Eating less and moving more should help you to lose weight and hence reduce your insulin resistance and your risks of type 2 diabetes. Even if you're not overweight, just moving more should reduce your insulin resistance and thus reduce your risks of type 2 diabetes.

Nevertheless, just as there are always going to be some people who can't lose weight no matter what they do, short of actual starvation, there are always going to be some people who get type 2 diabetes no matter what they do. Their genetic tendency is simply too great for environmental influences to have a large enough effect.

If you happen to be one of these people, don't blame yourself. It's bad enough to get the disease without having to deal with guilt. Don't let your health care professionals blame you either. If they hint, or say outright, that being overweight and getting diabetes is all your fault because you're lazy or lack willpower, find other doctors.

When you see comments in the media that type 2 diabetes is completely preventable, remember that this is not always true. Most cases can be postponed until old age and sometimes even prevented by continually working hard to eat no more than you need and to exercise as much as possible. But not all. In the Diabetes Prevention Program trials I mentioned earlier, diet and exercise reduced the incidence of type 2 diabetes in prediabetic people by 58 percent. That's certainly significant. But what people forget is that it *didn't* work for everyone. It's possible those who dieted and exercised and still got diabetes didn't work quite as hard at it. It's also possible they just had a bigger genetic tendency to get the disease.

Diabetes is very uncommon in non-Westernized people, but it still occurs occasionally. What is happening today is that instead of 0.5 percent of such people getting type 2 diabetes, now 15 percent or 25 percent or even 50 percent of them develop the disease.

Understanding that there are some things beyond your control may help you deal with the complexities of this disease if it runs in your family. Do what you can to prevent it. But if your efforts fail, don't get mired down in guilt. It's probably not your fault.

RESOURCES

Organizations offering further information about diabetes

American Diabetes Association
1701 North Beauregard Street
Alexandria, VA 22311
800-342-2383 (800-DIABETES)
www.diabetes.org/

Joslin Diabetes Center
One Joslin Place
Boston, MA 02115
617-732-2440
www.joslin.harvard.edu/

National Diabetes Information Clearinghouse
1 Information Way
Bethesda, MD 20892-3560
800-860-8747; 301-654-3327
www.niddk.nih.gov/health/diabetes/ndic.htm

The National Diabetes Information Clearinghouse offers a lot of free publications on all aspects of diabetes, many in both English and Spanish. Ask for their publications list.

Sources of hard-to-find low-glycemic index foods

Native Seeds/SEARCH
526 N. Fourth Avenue
Tuscon, AZ 85705
www.nativeseeds.org

Native Seeds/SEARCH sells unusual low–glycemic index desert foods such as tepary beans, mesquite flour, and nopal cactus, as well as seeds so you can grow your own. Ask for their catalog.

Pinewoods Products
13466 Four Mile Level Road
Gowanda, NY 14070
716-532-5241

Pinewoods sells low–glycemic index Iroquois white corn in the form of roasted white corn flour, hulled hominy, and tamal flour (hulled hominy flour). This is the type of corn that was originally grown in the Americas. Our common sweet corn is a higher–glycemic index version of the original corn.

Sources of glycemic load information

http://www.mendosa.com/gilists.htm
This is a simplified version of the paper cited next and may be the easiest to use.

Foster-Powell, Kaye, Susanna H. A. Holt, Janette C. Brand-Miller. International table of glycemic index and glycemic load values: 2002. *American Journal of Clinical Nutrition.* 76 (2002):5–56.

This is the most complete version of current glycemic load information and includes serving sizes, references, and the types of subjects used to determine the values.

Brand-Miller, Jennie, Thomas M. S. Wolever, Stephen Colagiuri, Kaye Foster-Powell. *The New Glucose Revolution.* New York: Marlowe, 2003.

This book is scheduled for publication in early 2003.

Some useful books about diabetes

American Diabetes Association. *American Diabetes Association Complete Guide to Diabetes*, 2nd ed. New York: Bantam Books, 2000.

The official ADA viewpoint of diabetes.

Beaser, Richard S., Joan V. C. Hill. *The Joslin Guide to Diabetes* (in both English and Spanish). New York: Simon & Schuster, 1995.

Diabetes information from the viewpoint of the Joslin Diabetes Center, one of the leading diabetes centers in the country.

Becker, Gretchen. *The First Year—Type 2 Diabetes.* New York: Marlowe, 2001.

A patient-oriented viewpoint of diabetes.

Books describing different diet approaches

Ideally, your way of eating will evolve to the point that you don't need to follow any rigid diet plan. You'll automatically choose small portions of a variety of tasty whole foods—with occasional splurges on special occasions. But it often helps to start out with a more structured approach.

There are many, many different diet books on the market. The following is only a small sample. If you can, go to a large bookstore and browse the various books until you find one that seems to address your needs. Look for something that explains as much of the science of the diet as you want to know, includes foods you like to eat, and has recipes that appeal to you.

Low-carbohydrate diet

Allan, Christian B., Wolfgang Lutz. *Life Without Bread*. Los Angeles: Keats Publishing, 2000.

> The diet consists of 72 grams of carbohydrate a day and as much of anything else as you want. No other rules. The authors claim that overweight children always lose weight on this diet, although adults may not. Rather than providing menus and recipes, most of the book consists of discussion of why this diet works.

Atkins, Robert C. *Dr. Atkins' New Diet Revolution,* rev. ed. New York: Avon, 2001.

> One of the classic low-carb diets. It doesn't discourage eating saturated fat and recommends a lot of supplements, especially the author's own brand.

Broadhurst, C. Leigh. *Diabetes: Prevention and Cure*. New York: Kensington Books, 1999.

> Discusses fats, antioxidants, chromium and other micronutrients, and medicinal plants. The diet emphasizes fresh vegetables and fruits, but also a lot of supplements and sports nutrition bars.

Eades, Michael R., Mary Dan Eades. *Protein Power*. New York: Bantam Books, 1997.

> Similar to the Atkins diet with useful tables showing the

carbohydrate content of foods when the fiber has been subtracted.

Ezrin, Calvin, Robert E. Kowalski: *The Type 2 Diabetes Diet Book*, 3rd rev. ed. New York: McGraw-Hill, 1999.
A spartan low-carb, low-fat diet.

Goldberg, Jack, Karen O'Mara. *GO-Diet*. Niles, Ill.: GO Corporation, 1999.
A low-carb diet that also emphasizes monounsaturated fat and fiber and says supplements aren't necessary.

Low-fat, high carbohydrate and fiber
McDougall, John A. *The McDougall Program for Maximum Weight Loss*. New York: Plume, 1995.
A vegetarian high-fiber diet.

Ornish, Dean. *Eat More, Weigh Less,* rev. ed. New York: Quill, 2000.
An extremely low-fat diet that emphasizes other lifestyle changes such as stress reduction and exercise as well.

Physicians Committee for Responsible Medicine. *Healthy Eating for Life to Prevent and Treat Diabetes*. New York: John Wiley, 2002.
A vegan whole-food diet along with some information about diabetes.

Low–glycemic index diet
Brand-Miller, Jennie, Johanna Burani, Kaye Foster-Powell. *The Glucose Revolution Life Plan*. New York: Marlowe, 1999.
An outline of the glycemic index principles by some of the authors of the classic work on the glycemic index, along with information about dietary fats and discussions of other diets.

Leighton, Steward H., Morrison C. Bethea, Sam S. Andrews, Luis A. Balart. *Sugar Busters!* New York: Ballantine, 1998.

One of the first American diets to adopt the glycemic index concept.

Montignac, Michel. *Eat Yourself Slim*. Michel Ange, 1999.

The French version of a low–glycemic index diet, translated and adapted for English readers.

Theories of dieting

Pool, Robert. *Fat—Fighting the Obesity Epidemic*. New York: Oxford University Press, 2001.

Calculating nutritional content

Pennington, Jean A. T. *Bowes & Church's Food Values of Portions Commonly Used,* 17th ed. Philadelphia: Lippincott Williams & Wilkins, 1998.

USDA Nutrient Database for Standard Reference online at *http://www.nal.usda.gov/fnic/cgi-bin/nut_search.pl*

Diet cookbooks

Most of the major diets have cookbooks to match their diet plans. I don't usually use cookbooks and haven't tried very many, but following are a couple that I think are especially good.

Low-carbohydrate cookbook

McCullough, Fran. *The Low-Carb Cookbook*. New York: Hyperion, 2001.

If you like good food and aren't afraid of unusual ingredients, you'll love this book. Everything I tried was delicious. If you're looking for one hundred ways to serve hamburger, you might prefer one of the many other low-carb cookbooks now on the market.

Low-fat cookbook

Goor, Ron, Nancy Goor. *Eater's Choice Low-Fat Cookbook.* Boston: Houghton Mifflin, 1999.

I've eaten Nancy's cooking and tried some of her recipes, and they're always delicious as well as creative.

Diabetic exchange diet cookbooks

Most "diabetic cookbooks" you find in bookstores follow the diabetic exchange system. There are a multitude of these cookbooks, for almost every taste. If you're interested in this approach, browse through as many as you can find and choose one that matches your tastes.

ABOUT THE AUTHOR

gretchen becker, a magna cum laude and Phi Beta Kappa graduate of Radcliffe College, is a writer and editor specializing in medical books and the author of *The First Year—Type 2 Diabetes*. She was diagnosed with type 2 diabetes in 1996 and is a longtime participant in several diabetes e-mail lists on the Internet. She lives on a small farm in Halifax, Vermont.